KU-025-058

Foreword

This book contains questions similar to those that may be found on state licensing exams for nail technology. It employs the multiple-choice type question, which has been widely adopted and approved by the majority of state licensing boards.

Groups of questions have been arranged under major subject areas. To get the maximum advantage when using this book, it is advisable that the review of subject matter takes place shortly after its classroom presentation.

This review book reflects advances in professional nail technology. It attempts to keep pace with, and insure a basic understanding of, sanitation, anatomy, physiology, and salon business applicable to the nail technician, client consultation guidelines, chemical safety in the nail salon, and basic manicuring and pedicuring procedures as well as some of the more advanced and creative aspects of the profession.

The book serves as an excellent guide for the student as well as for the experienced nail technician. It provides a reliable standard against which professionals can measure their knowledge, understanding, and abilities.

Furthermore, these reviews will help students and professionals alike to gain a more thorough understanding of the full scope of their work as they review practical performance skills and related theory. They will increase their ability to evaluate new products and procedures and to be better qualified professionals for dealing with the needs of their clients.

Warrington Collegiate - Learning
Resouce Centre

A107399

Milady Standard
Nail
Exam Review

CENGAGE
Learning

Australia • Brazil • Mexico • Singapore • United Kingdom • United States

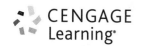

CENGAGE Learning®

Exam Review for Milady Standard Nail Technology, Seventh Edition

Milady

Executive Director, Milady: Sandra Bruce

Product Director: Corina Santoro

Product Manager: Philip I. Mandl

Product Assistant: Mary Lates

Director, Marketing & Training: Gerard McAvey

Community Manager: Matthew McGuire

Senior Production Director: Wendy Troeger

Production Manager: Sherondra Thedford

Senior Content Project Manager: Nina Tucciarelli

Senior Art Director: Benj Gleeksman

Cover image: © Henry Arden/ Cultura/Corbis

© 2015 Milady, a part of Cengage Learning

ALL RIGHTS RESERVED. No part of this work covered by the copyright herein may be reproduced, transmitted, stored, or used in any form or by any means graphic, electronic, or mechanical, including but not limited to photocopying, recording, scanning, digitizing, taping, Web distribution, information networks, or information storage and retrieval systems, except as permitted under Section 107 or 108 of the 1976 United States Copyright Act, without the prior written permission of the publisher.

For product information and technology assistance, contact us at **Cengage Learning Customer & Sales Support, 1-800-354-9706**

For permission to use material from this text or product, submit all requests online at **www.cengage.com/permissions**. Further permissions questions can be emailed to **permissionrequest@cengage.com**

Library of Congress Control Number: 2013954496

ISBN-13: 978-1-285-08054-3

ISBN-10: 1-285-08054-8

Milady
5 Maxwell Drive
Clifton Park, NY 12065-2919
USA

Cengage Learning is a leading provider of customized learning solutions with office locations around the globe, including Singapore, the United Kingdom, Australia, Mexico, Brazil, and Japan. Locate your local office at: **international.cengage.com/region**

Cengage Learning products are represented in Canada by Nelson Education, Ltd.

For your lifelong learning solutions, visit **milady.cengage.com**

Purchase any of our products at your local college store or at our preferred online store **www.cengagebrain.com**

Visit our corporate website at **cengage.com**.

Notice to the Reader

Publisher does not warrant or guarantee any of the products described herein or perform any independent analysis in connection with any of the product information contained herein. Publisher does not assume, and expressly disclaims, any obligation to obtain and include information other than that provided to it by the manufacturer. The reader is expressly warned to consider and adopt all safety precautions that might be indicated by the activities described herein and to avoid all potential hazards. By following the instructions contained herein, the reader willingly assumes all risks in connection with such instructions. The publisher makes no representations or warranties of any kind, including but not limited to, the warranties of fitness for particular purpose or merchantability, nor are any such representations implied with respect to the material set forth herein, and the publisher takes no responsibility with respect to such material. The publisher shall not be liable for any special, consequential, or exemplary damages resulting, in whole or part, from the readers' use of, or reliance upon, this material.

Printed in the United States of America
1 2 3 4 5 6 7 18 17 16 15 14

Milady Standard
Nail Technology Exam Review

Part I: Chapter Review Tests

CHAPTER 1: HISTORY AND CAREER OPPORTUNITIES

1. Which term refers to the art and science of beautifying
   and improving the nails and skin of the hands and feet?
   a. cosmetology
   b. nail technology
   c. esthetics
   d. manicuring   ____

2. In what year was the first successful nail lacquer brand
   marketed?
   a. 1910
   b. 1925
   c. 1932
   d. 1940   ____

3. Who were the first people to use cosmetics to prepare
   the deceased for burial?
   a. The Egyptians
   b. The Greeks
   c. The Romans
   d. The Chinese   ____

4. Ancient Egyptians used _____ to stain their hair
   and nails a rich, warm red.
   a. camel blood
   b. rose petals
   c. henna paste
   d. crushed insects   ____

5. In which ancient cultures did military commanders stain
   their nails and lips in matching colors before important
   battles?
   a. Chinese and Greek
   b. Egyptian and Roman
   c. Greek and Roman
   d. Chinese and Egyptian   ____

6. Which practice was closely tied to social status during
   the Chou Dynasty?
   a. Nail tinting
   b. Hair tinting
   c. Lip tinting
   d. Cheek tinting   ____

7. In which ancient culture could commoners be put to
   death for wearing the royal nail colors?
   a. Egyptian
   b. Roman
   c. Chinese
   d. Greek   ____

8. The ancient Greeks made lavish use of perfumes
   and cosmetics for grooming, medicinal purposes,
   and _____.
   a. religious rites
   b. burial rites
   c. social rites
   d. family events   ____

9. Which ancient culture built elaborate baths and developed excellent methods of dressing the hair?
   a. The Romans
   c. The Egyptians
   b. The Greeks
   d. The Chinese
   _____

10. When preparing for battle, what color did Greek soldiers often apply to their lips and nails?
   a. Red
   c. Brown
   b. Black
   d. Blue
   _____

11. Where did ancient Greek women apply kohl?
   a. To their cheeks
   c. To their hair
   b. To their eyes
   d. To their nails
   _____

12. What did ancient Greek women apply to their lips to add color?
   a. Ground cinnabar
   c. Henna paste
   b. Insect blood
   d. Lead powder
   _____

13. The Roman philosopher Plautus is credited with comparing a woman without paint (cosmetics) to _____.
   a. music without instruments
   c. food without salt
   b. a day without sunshine
   d. life without music
   _____

14. If you were a noblewoman in ancient Rome, you would color your hair _____ to indicate your class status.
   a. brown
   c. blond
   b. black
   d. red
   _____

15. In ancient Rome, it was common for both men and women to add color to their nails using a mixture of sheep blood and _____.
   a. powder
   c. fat
   b. roots
   d. bark
   _____

16. Which period immediately followed the Middle Ages?
   a. The Roman Empire
   c. The Ice Age
   b. The Victorian Age
   d. The Renaissance
   _____

17. During the _____, the use of highly colored preparations for the lips, cheeks, eyes, and nails was discouraged.
   a. Middle Ages
   c. Roman Empire
   b. Victorian Age
   d. Renaissance
   _____

18. Archaeological digs have uncovered cosmetic tools from the Renaissance period, including nail cleaners, some doubling as _____, made of bone or metal in a wide variety of designs.
   a. nail files
   c. eye cleaners
   b. ear scoops
   d. hair brushes
   _____

19. Victorian women _____ to induce natural lip color.
    a. applied rouge
    c. applied lip stains
    b. bit their lips
    d. applied natural ingredients   _____

20. The onset of _____ led to a new prosperity in the United States, during which all forms of beauty began to follow trends.
    a. World War I
    c. industrialization
    b. the Great Depression
    d. assembly lines   _____

21. The first noncaking, non-cracking makeup was marketed to movie stars _____.
    a. Max Factor
    c. Mary Kay
    b. Charles Revson
    d. Charles Graf   _____

22. In 1910, Flowery Manicure Products introduced the first modern-style _____.
    a. nail polish
    c. nail wrap
    b. emery board
    d. artificial nail   _____

23. Who introduced the first mass-marketed nail lacquers?
    a. Yves Rocher
    c. Madam C. J. Walker
    b. Paul Mitchell
    d. Charles Revson   _____

24. Jean Harlow and _____ helped glamorize the hip new nail lacquer trend in the 1930s by wearing matching colors on her fingers and toes.
    a. Gloria Swanson
    c. Marilyn Monroe
    b. Elizabeth Taylor
    d. Lillian Gish   _____

25. Shiny lips came into vogue for the first time in the _____ when women began applying petroleum jelly over their lipstick.
    a. 1920s
    c. 1940s
    b. 1930s
    d. 1950s   _____

26. The 1950s saw the introduction of tube mascara, improved hair care and nail products, and the boom of _____.
    a. artificial nail enhancements
    c. opaque paint
    b. monthly hair care appointments
    d. weekly manicure appointments   _____

27. When did hot oil manicures first become the ultimate luxury in nail and hand care?
    a. The 1950s
    c. The 1970s
    b. The 1960s
    d. The 1980s   _____

28. Which of the following is credited with establishing the biweekly nail maintenance appointment?
    a. Fiberglass wraps
    b. Juliette wraps
    c. Silk wraps
    d. UV gel nail services ＿＿＿＿

29. In the 1960s, where did the nails from nail technicians' "nail banks" typically come from?
    a. Hospital patients
    b. Friends and family
    c. Their clients
    d. Plastics manufacturers ＿＿＿＿

30. When were the first monomer liquid and polymer powder nail services offered by nail technicians?
    a. The 1960s
    b. The 1970s
    c. The 1980s
    d. The 1990s ＿＿＿＿

31. Who invented the first Ridgefiller?
    a. Jeff Pink
    b. Charles Revson
    c. Jean Harlow
    d. Yves Rocher ＿＿＿＿

32. When did the use of spray guns to apply monomer liquid nail colors become common?
    a. The 1970s
    b. The 1980s
    c. The 1990s
    d. The 1960s ＿＿＿＿

33. The 1990s ushered in a huge resurgence in ＿＿＿＿＿＿ and pedicure services.
    a. plain manicure
    b. artificial nail enhancements
    c. hot oil manicure
    d. natural manicure ＿＿＿＿

34. In the 1960s, detached nail tips were reaffixed with ＿＿＿＿＿＿.
    a. model airplane glue
    b. wood glue
    c. instant resin
    d. nail paste ＿＿＿＿

35. Which part of the nail did nail technicians commonly leave free of polish in the 1950s?
    a. The tip
    b. The side edges
    c. The moon
    d. The free edge ＿＿＿＿

36. One notable achievement of the twentieth century included the fact that nail technicians had ＿＿＿＿＿＿.
    a. more clients than ever
    b. unprecedented career choices
    c. made more money
    d. less regulatory oversight ＿＿＿＿

37. A new, opaque paint being produced for the automobile industry inspired the introduction of the first mass-marketed ＿＿＿＿＿＿.
    a. lipsticks
    b. mascaras
    c. nail lacquers
    d. makeup ＿＿＿＿

38. In the 1960s, nail technicians reaffixed detached nail tips and reinforced them with what?
   a. Thin paper strips
   b. Thick fabric strips
   c. Thin sewing thread
   d. Thin strands of cotton _____

39. Another notable beauty industry achievement of the twentieth century included nail polish becoming _____.
   a. softer and lighter
   b. brighter and thicker
   c. darker and heavier
   d. safer and longer-lasting _____

40. In the early twenty-first century, UV gel enhancements _____.
   a. are less and less popular
   b. grow by leaps and bounds
   c. require more curing
   d. last less than two weeks _____

41. Modern nail polish formulations embody chip- and _____-resistant characteristics.
   a. smear
   b. lift
   c. fade
   d. streak _____

42. Modern manicuring implements now incorporate _____ designs and enhanced workmanship.
   a. state-of-the-art
   b. simple
   c. more complex
   d. ergonomic _____

43. A regular nail technician in a traditional salon can expect to do all but which of the following?
   a. Work with UV gel nail products
   b. Work under the supervision of a physician
   c. Provide manicures and pedicures
   d. Offer silk nail wrap services _____

44. To become a medical nail technician, you are required to take specialty course and complete an internship under the direction of a _____ physician.
   a. physician's assistant
   b. nurse practitioner
   c. registered nurse
   d. podiatrist _____

45. Which of these services is commonly offered by day spas, but not full-service salons?
   a. Body services
   b. Hair services
   c. Skin services
   d. Nail services _____

CHAPTER 2: LIFE SKILLS

1. The salon is a highly social atmosphere that requires
    _____ and excellent people skills.
    a. frequent events
    b. lively music
    c. strong self-discipline
    d. television monitors   ____

2. The ability to deal with difficult clients, coworkers, and
    even friends comes from having _____.
    a. positive goals
    b. assertiveness skills
    c. average communication
        skills
    d. well-developed life skills   ____

3. Having good life skills builds _____, which helps
    you achieve your goals.
    a. high self-esteem
    b. strong assertiveness
    c. a winning personality
    d. leadership responsibility   ____

4. Self-esteem is based on inner strength and begins
    with trusting your ability to _____.
    a. communicate with others
    b. reach your goals
    c. become popular
    d. handle clients effectively   ____

5. _____ or negative thoughts can work against
    your ability to succeed.
    a. Unsure behavior
    b. Vigorous exercise
    c. Self-critical
    d. Frequent naps   ____

6. To achieve success it is important to make a point
    of relating to others with a conscious feeling of _____.
    a. respect
    b. criticism
    c. admiration
    d. confidence   ____

7. Three bad habits that can keep you from maintaining
    peak performance include lack of a game plan, seeking
    perfectionism, and _____.
    a. annual planning
    b. making mistakes
    c. failing to prioritize
    d. procrastination   ____

8. One recommended way to keep your energy up
    is to _____.
    a. avoid spending a lot
        of time with family
        and friends
    b. eat, sleep, and drink
        beauty
    c. have hobbies and enjoy
        recreational activities
    d. take on as many
        responsibilities as
        possible   ____

9. One guideline for success suggests that you practice doing whatever helps you maintain _____.
   a. an elevated ego
   b. a positive self-image
   c. a friendly approach
   d. a comfortable demeanor _____

10. Procrastination may be a symptom of _____.
    a. a characteristic of good study habits
    b. an unhealthy compulsion to do things perfectly
    c. a result of exceptional organization
    d. a symptom of taking on too much _____

11. Perfectionism is _____.
    a. a characteristic of good study habits
    b. an unhealthy compulsion to do things perfectly
    c. a result of exceptional organization
    d. a symptom of taking on too much _____

12. Having a game plan is the conscious act of _____.
    a. randomly accepting life
    b. planning today
    c. being a free spirit
    d. planning your life _____

13. _____ involves knowing what you want to achieve and keeping yourself on track so that you do eventually achieve your goal.
    a. Self-management
    b. Personal desire
    c. Personal motivation
    d. Self-indulgence _____

14. Which of the following blocks the creative mind from exploring ideas and discovering solutions to challenges?
    a. Analysis
    b. Motivation
    c. Criticism
    d. Familial support _____

15. One of the recommended ways to manage your own success is to _____.
    a. criticize yourself for your mistakes
    b. tap into your own creativity
    c. strike out and work alone.
    d. look to others for motivation _____

16. To succeed in life, you need a well-thought-out sense of purpose and a _____.
    a. balanced checkbook
    b. reason for being
    c. memorized goals
    d. sense of adventure _____

17. How long should your personal mission statement be?
    a. A brief summary
    b. One or two sentences
    c. One or two paragraphs
    d. One or two pages _____

18. For reinforcement, keep a copy of your mission statement _____.
    a. where you can see and read it daily
    b. in a secure place, such as a safe
    c. in a file with your financial documents
    d. in a file with your educational transcripts   _____

19. What is the primary purpose of goal setting?
    a. To outline your daily activities
    b. To help increase your self-esteem
    c. To identify the best places for employment
    d. To help you decide what you want to achieve in life   _____

20. Which of the following is *not* a key question you should ask to determine if your goal-setting plan is a good one?
    a. Am I always open to finding better ways of putting my plan into practice?
    b. Is goal-setting a practical way to spend my time at this point in my career?
    c. Is the information I need to reach my goals readily available?
    d. Would I be willing to seek out a mentor to enhance my learning?   _____

21. What are the two basic types of goals?
    a. Primary and secondary
    b. Relevant and irrelevant
    c. Long-term and short-term
    d. Professional and personal   _____

22. Which of the following is an example of a long-term goal?
    a. I will work my way up to salon manager within 3 to 5 years.
    b. I will finish the semester with at least a 3.5 GPA.
    c. I will get a perfect score on my next exam.
    d. I will devote the next week to sending out copies of my resume.   _____

23. The important thing to remember about goal setting is to _____.
    a. lock yourself into a rigid plan
    b. have a plan and reexamine it often
    c. avoid adjusting goals and action plans
    d. focus on what feels good today   _____

24. Time management experts agree that all of us have _____.
    a. an inner organizer
    b. artistic talent
    c. a strong drive to succeed
    d. a working system   _____

25. When asked to take on more work than you can handle, it is recommended that you _____.
   a. agree to take the work on and do your best to get it done
   b. state that you are not sure if you can get the work done
   c. agree, then apologize later for not getting the work done
   d. say "no" firmly but kindly and mean it   _____

26. Time management experts recommend that you give yourself some downtime whenever you are frustrated, worried, feeling guilty about something, or _____.
   a. can fit it in   c. feel optimistic
   b. nervous   d. overwhelmed   _____

27. When you practice deep breathing, how many breaths does it typically take to restore your balance?
   a. Just one   c. 5–10
   b. 2–3   d. 15–20   _____

28. Which of these is not a practice recommended by time management experts?
   a. Plan your schedule around the times of day you are most and least energetic.
   b. Fill every slot in your schedule with some kind of task, no matter how small.
   c. Avoid neglecting physical activity.
   d. Understand the value of to-do lists for the day and week.   _____

29. If your mind tends to wander in class, you should _____.
   a. write down key words and phrases
   b. spend lecture time rereading the chapter being discussed
   c. attend class only on days when exams are given
   d. hire a tutor to help you learn the material   _____

30. Before you begin studying, you should find a comfortable, quiet spot with sufficient lighting and _____.
   a. a place to recline
   b. loud music to block distractions
   c. your smartphone and other communication devices
   d. all the tools you need such as books, pens, paper, and computer   _____

31. When studying, it is recommended that you study one chapter section at a time, noting key words and phrases, and _____.
   a. politely accept interruptions as they occur
   b. test yourself on each section to ensure comprehension
   c. refrain from highlighting the material
   d. forge ahead even when you can no longer focus   _____

32. Which term refers to the moral principles by which we
    live and work?
    a. Integrity   c. Ethics
    b. Self-image   d. Perfectionism   _____

33. When you make sure that your behavior and actions
    match your values, you maintain your _____.
    a. integrity   c. ability to communicate
    b. discretion   d. personality   _____

34. By not sharing your personal problems with clients
    and never breaching confidentiality you demonstrate
    that you are _____.
    a. independent   c. self-centered
    b. discreet   d. communicative   _____

35. Practicing ethics in the salon every day is manifested
    by being _____, courteous, and sincere.
    a. timely   c. hygienic
    b. happy   d. honest   _____

36. The ingredients of a healthy, well-developed attitude
    include all *BUT* which of the following?
    a. Tact and diplomacy   c. Striving for perfection
    b. Emotional stability   d. Pleasing tone of voice _____

37. To be truly helpful to others, you must remember to take
    time every single day to _____.
    a. take care of yourself   c. revise your schedule
    b. practice your skills   d. reexamine your goals   _____

38. In order to help people understand your position,
    it can be a good thing to be _____.
    a. aggressive   c. antagonistic
    b. assertive   d. a procrastinator   _____

39. Diplomacy involves being _____, which is the
    ability to deliver truthful, even sometimes critical or
    difficult messages in a kind way.
    a. arrogant   c. tactful
    b. apprehensive   d. inconsiderate   _____

40. Having _____ helps you deliver your words
    more pleasantly.
    a. a positive attitude   c. a skilled mentor
    b. a well-defined set of goals d. an aggressive personality _____

41. A person's personality includes inborn characteristics, attitudes, and _____.
   a. appearance
   b. actions
   c. behavioral traits
   d. moods
   _____

42. Learning how to handle a confrontation and being able to share how you feel without going overboard are indicators of _____.
   a. talent
   b. creativity
   c. maturity
   d. perseverance
   _____

43. Sensitivity is a combination of understanding, empathy, and _____.
   a. pity
   b. acceptance
   c. sympathy
   d. willingness
   _____

44. Values and goals are _____.
   a. inborn characteristics
   b. acquired as a person moves through life
   c. irrelevant aspects of one's personality
   d. unchangeable once acquired
   _____

45. To be receptive means to be interested in other people and _____.
   a. be responsive to their opinions, feelings, and ideas
   b. refuse to consider the beliefs and values of others
   c. listen primarily to only what interests you
   d. have excellent communication skills
   _____

CHAPTER 3: YOUR PROFESSIONAL IMAGE

1. When your appearance and the way that you conduct yourself are in harmony with the beauty business, your chances of being successful increase _____.
   a. slightly
   b. dramatically
   c. overtime
   d. gradually _____

2. One weak moment of _____ right before performing a service because you did not plan ahead could spell disaster.
   a. calling a friend
   b. posting on Facebook
   c. texting a colleague
   d. drinking coffee _____

3. Most clients will _____ if you smell offensive, and they will not likely return for another service.
   a. say nothing
   b. tell you discreetly
   c. tell you bluntly
   d. cancel the appointment _____

4. Working as a _____ means you must be extremely meticulous about your hygiene.
   a. concerned citizen
   b. computer programmer
   c. nail technician
   d. technical writer _____

5. Which of these items should be kept in your hygiene pack?
   a. Toothbrush
   b. Teeth whitener
   c. Lipstick
   d. Gum _____

6. Good personal hygiene habits include washing your hands throughout the day as required, including _____.
   a. before each service
   b. before applying nail polish
   c. after filing a client's nails
   d. after applying nail polish _____

7. Which of these items is not typically part of a hygiene pack?
   a. Sanitizing hand wipes
   b. Dental floss
   c. Shampoo
   d. Mouthwash _____

8. The professional nail technician should brush and floss his or her teeth and use _____ throughout the day as needed.
   a. lotion
   b. antiseptic
   c. fragrance
   d. mouthwash _____

9. If you must smoke cigarettes, do not smoke _____.
   a. at home
   b. during work hours
   c. in your car
   d. during social events _____

10. If you smoke during your lunch break, brush your teeth, use mouthwash, and wash your hands afterward to avoid _____.
    a. premature aging
    b. gum disease
    c. dry mouth
    d. an offensive lingering smell   _____

11. As a beauty professional, it is recommended that you change your style: _____
    a. frequently.   c. twice a year.
    b. annually.   d. as your mood suggests.   _____

12. Many salon owners and managers view appearance and poise as being _____ technical knowledge and skills.
    a. less important than   c. just as important as
    b. more important than   d. not relevant to   _____

13. In addition to being free of dirt, it is important that your clothes be _____.
    a. stain free   c. new
    b. colorful   d. expensive   _____

14. You should always put _____ first in every aspect of your work.
    a. the task at hand   c. your health
    b. your potential earnings   d. the salon's bottom line _____

15. To help protect your clothes from dirt and stains, you should invest in _____ to wear at work.
    a. a pair of coveralls   c. a pair of scrubs
    b. an apron or smock   d. Scotch-guarded clothing   _____

16. It is recommended that you only wear perfume _____.
    a. after work   c. after smoking
    b. before work   d. throughout the day   _____

17. Your professional image is the impression you project through both your _____.
    a. thoughts and attitude
    b. attitude and personality
    c. outward appearance and professional conduct
    d. appearance and social conduct   _____

18. The best way to ensure that you are dressed for success is to "tune in" to _____.
    a. your innermost desires
    b. your career goals
    c. the weather and environment
    d. the salon's culture and clientele

19. When shopping for work clothes, you should primarily think about _____.
    a. whether you are getting a good bargain
    b. how you would look in them while performing client services
    c. whether they enhance your figure to the maximum
    d. how long they will be in style

20. To a large degree, your clothing should _____.
    a. reflect the fashions of the season
    b. be completely unique and unexpected
    c. focus on comfort over appearance
    d. be replaced every two to three weeks

21. It is generally a good idea to make sure that your clothing is clean, _____, and stylish.
    a. colorful
    b. dry-clean only
    c. washable
    d. functional

22. Which of these jewelry items is least appropriate for the typical salon?
    a. A pair of stud earrings
    b. A thin rope necklace
    c. A loose, jingly bracelet
    d. A band-style ring

23. Your shoes should have a low heel and _____.
    a. offer good support
    b. have a soft sole
    c. have a tight fit
    d. have a loose fit

24. When should female technicians wear makeup at work?
    a. Never
    b. Always
    c. Occasionally
    d. As directed

25. Good physical posture, an even gait, and careful movements are very important parts of your _____.
    a. physical strength
    b. personal agility
    c. personality and attitude
    d. physical presentation

26. _____ can put a great deal of stress on your neck, shoulders, back, and legs.
    a. Standing erectly
    b. Jogging regularly
    c. Walking slowly
    d. Sitting improperly ____

27. Stress on the body can cause strain and/or _____.
    a. lethargy
    b. illness
    c. injury
    d. energy ____

28. As you work, your neck should be _____.
    a. elongated and balanced above the shoulders
    b. bent over client
    c. leaning toward your dominant hand
    d. leaning away from your dominant hand ____

29. As you work, you should keep your chest _____.
    a. up and in
    b. out and up
    c. down and in
    d. relaxed ____

30. You should keep your back _____ as you work.
    a. curved
    b. bent
    c. straight
    d. turned ____

31. Your _____ should be pulled in so that it is flat while you work.
    a. back
    b. neck
    c. chest
    d. abdomen ____

32. As a professional nail technician, an extremely important element of _____ is having well-groomed hair, skin, and nails.
    a. professional posture
    b. your image
    c. personal deportment
    d. your career goals ____

33. Busy nail technicians are susceptible to problems of the hands, wrists, and _____.
    a. elbows
    b. chest
    c. feet
    d. shoulders ____

34. An understanding of _____ can help prevent stress on the body as you work.
    a. ergonomics
    b. eczema
    c. cryogenics
    d. macroeconomics ____

35. One goal of ergonomics is to make workplace tools more safe and _____.
    a. attractive
    b. economical
    c. efficient
    d. flexible ____

16

36. In general, ergonomics attempts to _____.
    a. fit the person to the job   c. accommodate different positions
    b. fit the job to the person   d. completely automate the salon   _____

37. An awareness of your body posture and _____, coupled with better work habits and proper tools and equipment, will enhance your health and comfort.
    a. weight   c. height
    b. activity   d. movements   _____

38. As you work, you should hold your elbows at no more than a _____ -degree angle away from your body for extended periods of time.
    a. 15   c. 60
    b. 25   d. 90   _____

39. As you work, your wrists should be _____ as much as possible.
    a. turned inward and extended   c. rested in a straight or neutral position
    b. bent and rigid   d. bent downward and relaxed   _____

40. You should have the client reach across the table to you during a manicure because this position is ergonomically correct for _____.
    a. both you and the client   c. the client
    b. neither you nor the client   d. you   _____

41. As you work, you should _____.
    a. use ergonomically designed implements   c. keeping your back and neck relaxed for comfort
    b. endure long periods of uninterrupted repetitive motions   d. avoid regular stretching exercises   _____

42. One measure that can be taken to prevent injury on the job is to break up the repetitiveness of motions used by including _____.
    a. regular stretching exercises   b. gripping implements tightly
    c. occasional bending and twisting   d. holding arms away from body   _____

43. Stressful, repetitive motions have a cumulative effect
    on the muscles and _____.
    a. skin   c. joints
    b. bones   d. tendons   ____

44. _____ allows you to get through the day feeling
    strong and doing your best work.
    a. Happiness   c. A good attitude
    b. Good posture   d. Exercise   ____

45. The term _____ refers to the daily maintenance
    of cleanliness achieved through healthful habits.
    a. professional image   c. physical presentation
    b. personal hygiene   d. professionalism   ____

CHAPTER 4: COMMUNICATING FOR SUCCESS

1. Effective human relations and communication skills build
   _____, accelerate professional growth, and help
   prevent misunderstandings in the workplace.
   a. strong values
   b. professional ethics
   c. stimulating conversations
   d. lasting client relationships   _____

2. When we feel secure, we act in a _____ manner.
   a. confident
   b. worried
   c. overwhelmed
   d. suspicious   _____

3. People who create conflict most likely feel _____.
   a. relaxed
   b. respected
   c. insecure
   d. secure   _____

4. A good way to handle the ups and downs of human relations
   is to _____.
   a. be inattentive
   b. believe in yourself
   c. talk more and listen less
   d. react instead of respond   _____

5. Which of the following is not one of the golden rules of
   human relations?
   a. Communicate from your head and problem-solve
      from your heart.
   b. See what happens when you ask for help instead of
      just reacting.
   c. Build shared goals by being a team player.
   d. Being right is different from acting righteous.   _____

6. Effective communication is defined as the act of _____.
   a. sending a message to another person or group
   b. receiving a message from another person or group
   c. repeating the speaker's words back in your own words
   d. sharing information between two people or groups   _____

7. When you meet a client for the first time, you need to
   be _____.
   a. very serious
   b. very instructive
   c. genuinely friendly
   d. strictly professional   _____

8. When a new client visits the salon for the first time, you should _____.
   a. assume a superior position
   b. introduce him/her only to other nail technicians
   c. take him/her on a quick tour of the facility
   d. assume that he/she already knows your name
   _____

9. When should you do the client consultation?
   a. Before the service starts
   b. During the service
   c. After the service
   d. On the phone prior to the appointment
   _____

10. You should perform a client consultation _____.
    a. only on the client's first visit to the salon
    b. to some degree, as part of every service
    c. about once a year if the client regularly visits the salon
    d. only when the client specifically requests one
    _____

11. The client consultation form is also sometimes called _____.
    a. a release statement
    b. a manager's questionnaire
    c. an employee evaluation form
    d. an intake form
    _____

12. The client consultation form typically does not ask _____.
    a. the client's age
    b. about prior nail services
    c. the client's goals for the salon visit
    d. about any chronic medical conditions
    _____

13. The client consultation form can best be described as a _____.
    a. list of salon policies.
    b. client questionnaire
    c. generalist of nail care tips
    d. list of nail services
    _____

14. How much time is it recommended that you set aside for the client consultation?
    a. 15–20 minutes
    b. 3–5 minutes
    c. 5–15 minutes
    d. 30 minutes
    _____

15. To help your client make choices that reflect a personal sense of style, it is recommended that you _____.
    a. research different fashion styles and determine which best suits the client
    b. use only the most current nail technologies
    c. master one popular style and apply to all clients
    d. perform the service style you are most comfortable with ___

16. A person who prefers classic styling in clothing would likely want a _____ with respect to her nails, makeup, and hair.
    a. simple and sophisticated look
    b. monochromatic nail polish
    c. no bright patterns or colors
    d. a look that demands greater attention ___

17. Which of these steps in the consultation process involves encouraging clients to flip through your photo collections to discuss what they like and why?
    a. Analyze the client's nails
    b. Make suggestions
    c. Show and tell
    d. Discuss upkeep and maintenance ___

18. Before the client gets to your station for the consultation you should _____.
    a. put out a variety of pictures showing different nail shapes, lengths, and designs
    b. mess it up a little so it looks like you have been very busy
    c. put away your photos of hand/foot models and nail charts
    d. put your portfolio and camera out of the way ___

19. A primary purpose of the client consultation is to have a conversation that will clue you in on his or her needs and _____.
    a. personal goals
    b. professional interests
    c. personal preferences
    d. family habits ___

20. When using the 10-step consultation method, what should you do next after discussing the client's personal preferences?
    a. Analyze the client's hands and fingertips.
    b. Have her look through photos and point out finished looks she likes.
    c. Make some style suggestions.
    d. Review the consultation form she filled out. ___

21. During the client consultation you should_____.
    a. refrain from suggesting   c. discuss the client's
       additional services   nail history
    b. try not to look directly   d. focus on the most
       at the client's nails   costly services   _____

22. Toward the end of the client consultation, you should counsel
    the client on the _____ associated with a given nail
    style or service as well as salon and home maintenance
    commitments needed to keep their nails looking their best
    at all times.
    a. work limitations   c. flamboyance
    b. noticeability   d. lifestyle limitations   _____

23. Your reactions to situations beyond your control, and your
    ability to _____ in the face of challenges, are critical
    to being successful in a people profession.
    a. stand up   c. control fear
    b. communicate   d. remain assertive   _____

24. Many salons set a limited amount of time that they allow
    a client to be late before they require them to reschedule.
    What is the common time limit?
    a. 15 minutes   c. 30 minutes
    b. 5 minutes   d. 45 minutes   _____

25. If your tardy client arrives and you have the time to take
    her without jeopardizing other clients' appointments, you
    should _____.
    a. refuse to take her and explain why
    b. refuse to take her without explaining why
    c. take her and act like there is not a problem
    d. take her but let her know why in a pleasant manner   _____

26. If you are running late and you know it will cause delays
    for a later client, it is recommended that you _____.
    a. hurry through the rest of your day and hope for the best
    b. have the client wait without explanation until you are ready
    c. have the receptionist call or text the client, explain
       the situation, and ask if she would like to reschedule
    d. call the client and cancel her appointment   _____

27. If you get involved in a scheduling mix-up, you should
    _____.
    a. be polite while arguing that you are correct
    b. be polite and refrain from arguing
    c. be assertive and argue that you are correct
    d. be aggressive but refrain from arguing   _____

28. If a client has a problem with the service and you cannot change what she dislikes, you should _____.
    a. honestly and tactfully explain why the problem cannot be fixed
    b. state that you cannot do what she wants, and return to other clients
    c. provide a compromised service in an attempt to please her
    d. apologize but firmly state it cannot be fixed ____

29. When faced with an unhappy client in a situation where you are unsure of what to do, it is recommended that you call on _____ or the salon manager for suggestions.
    a. a more experienced nail technician
    c. the newest trainee
    b. the salon owner
    d. another client ____

30. Why is it best to avoid the use of slang?
    a. It makes one appear uneducated.
    c. It may frustrate your clients.
    b. It is always against business policy.
    d. The same word can have a different meaning across cultures. ____

31. Mutual respect, which transforms a good nail technician into a _____ and colleague, naturally follows.
    a. well-known technician
    c. popular individual
    c. likable person
    d. trusted advisor ____

32. Always remember that _____ is the best relationship builder.
    a. laughing
    c. playing
    b. listening
    d. debating ____

33. When interacting with your coworkers, it is recommended that you _____.
    a. take sides when coworkers are arguing
    b. be honest even if it means being insensitive
    c. seek help from someone you respect when you are at odds with a coworker
    d. freely share details about your private life ____

34. Regardless of whether or not you like someone, your colleagues are professionals who deserve _____.
    a. your opinion
    c. total happiness
    b. career success
    d. your respect ____

35. The salon manager is generally the person with the most responsibility regarding the _____.
    a. salon's overall operation
    b. effectiveness of the telephone system
    c. front desk management
    d. inventory and supplies

36. When interacting with the salon manager, you should _____.
    a. try to minimize your mistakes
    b. discuss your colleagues
    c. be open to constructive criticism
    d. assume that a problem exists

37. A periodic review of an employee's behaviors and activities important to the salon is called _____.
    a. a consultation
    b. an employee evaluation
    c. an annual meeting
    d. an advisory session

38. Many beauty professionals do not take advantage of the crucial communication opportunity with their supervisor to discuss their _____.
    a. future advancements
    b. requests for policy changes
    c. personal hobbies
    d. observations of coworkers

39. At the end of an evaluation performance review meeting, _____.
    a. question the supervisor's observations
    b. begin discussions regarding pay
    c. thank the manager for the feedback and guidance
    d. invite the manager out for lunch

40. As the time for your review draws near, it is recommended that you _____.
    a. ask about possible promotions
    b. ask when you might be getting a raise
    c. perform a self-evaluation of your performance
    d. ask your manager about continuing education

41. A fundamental factor in human relations involves a person's sense of _____.
    a. security
    b. success
    c. accomplishment
    d. purpose

42. When you believe in yourself, you trust your judgment,
_____, and stick to what you believe is right.
   a. seek your goals   c. pursue happiness
   b. follow your dreams   d. uphold your values   _____

43. You can communicate through words, voice inflections,
_____, body language, or visual tools.
   a. thoughts   c. facial expressions
   b. dreams   d. mechanical tools   _____

44. Clients are coming to you for services and paying for your
expertise, which means you need to _____ every
time they come to see you.
   a. court them   c. challenge them
   b. change them   d. assume their loyalty   _____

45. Clients with a dramatic style generally _____.
   a. choose nail designs that   c. are less open to trying
      demand greater attention   new products
   b. choose nail designs that   d. dislike having additional
      allow for fewer options   services, such as nail art _____

CHAPTER 5: INFECTION CONTROL: PRINCIPLES AND PRACTICES

1. A mechanical process using soap and water or detergent and water to remove dirt, debris, and many disease-causing germs is known as _____.
   a. sanitizing
   b. disinfecting
   c. cleaning
   d. sterilizing _____

2. A chemical process used to reduce the number of disease-causing germs on surfaces to a safe level is known as _____.
   a. sanitizing
   b. disinfecting
   c. cleaning
   d. sterilizing _____

3. A chemical process that uses specific products to destroy organisms on nonporous surfaces is known as _____.
   a. sanitizing
   b. disinfecting
   c. cleaning
   d. sterilizing _____

4. Regulations prohibit nail technicians from _____ the living skin and from removing callused skin, warts, corns, and in-grown toenails.
   a. filing and buffing
   b. sloughing and scrubbing
   c. scraping and smoothing
   d. cutting or puncturing _____

5. OSHA stands for _____.
   a. Organization of Safety and Health Administration
   b. Oversight Section for Health Administration
   c. Occupational Safety and Health Administration
   d. Occupational Safety and Health Association _____

6. OSHA was created as part of the _____ to regulate and enforce standards to protect employees in the workplace.
   a. U.S. Department of Defense
   b. U.S. Department of Labor
   c. U.S. Department of Education
   d. U.S. Department of Employment _____

7. Prior to 2012, chemical manufacturers and importers were required to assess the potential hazards associated with their products by publishing _____.
   a. Material Safety Data Sheets
   b. Manufacturer Safety Data Sheets
   c. Material Surety Data Support
   d. Manufacturer Safety Data Support _____

8. In 2012, OSHA agreed to comply with the Globally Harmonized System of Classification and Labeling of Chemicals System (GHS) which requires the use of a standard-format called _____ (SDS) to replace the MSDS.
   a. Safety Data Support
   b. Surety Data Support
   c. Safety Data Sheets
   d. Safety Data Standards   ____

9. The SDS contains _____ categories of information.
   a. 10
   b. 12
   c. 14
   d. 16   ____

10. As part of the SDS categories, first-aid measures include important symptoms and effects as well as _____.
   a. product use
   b. required treatment
   c. use restrictions
   d. containment and cleanup   ____

11. As part of the SDS categories, handling and storage lists precautions for safe handling and storage, including _____.
   a. incompatibilities
   b. ingredients
   c. reactions
   d. identifiers   ____

12. As part of the SDS categories, toxicology information includes routes of exposure, related symptoms, and _____.
   a. safe handling and storage
   b. acute and chronic effects
   c. exposure and protection
   d. restrictions on transportation   ____

13. Either OSHA or, in some cases, state board inspectors can _____ if SDSs are not available during regular business hours.
   a. close the salon
   b. arrest the salon owner
   c. issue a fine to the salon
   d. revoke the salon license   ____

14. A disease that is caused by bacteria that are transmitted by coughing or sneezing is known as _____.
   a. tuberculosis
   b. fungal disease
   c. pneumonia
   d. virus   ____

15. It is against federal law to use any disinfecting product contrary to its _____.
   a. ingredients
   b. packaging
   c. intended use
   d. labeling   ____

16. A microscopic organism that normally exists in low concentrations in tap water that has been known to cause serious skin infections on legs after pedicures is _____.
    a. mesothelioma
    c. Methicillin-resistant Staphylococcus aureus
    b. Mycobacterium fortuitum
    d. bacilli ____

17. Laws are written by both federal and state legislatures to determine the _____ for a license holder and to establish guidelines for regulatory agencies to make rules.
    a. application requirements
    c. dress code
    b. scope of practice
    d. license renewal requirements ____

18. The invasion of body tissues by disease-causing pathogens is known as _____.
    a. a virus
    c. an infection
    b. an irritation
    d. a disease ____

19. The methods used to eliminate or reduce the transmission of infectious organisms are called _____.
    a. transmission control
    c. organism control
    b. infection reduction
    d. infection control ____

20. To determine the nature of a disease, such as a nail disease, from its symptoms is to _____ it.
    a. diagnose
    c. analyze
    b. assess
    d. evaluate ____

21. Disinfectants used in salons must be bactericidal, fungicidal, and _____.
    a. microcidal
    c. virucidal
    b. pathocidal
    d. germicidal ____

22. All of the following is true about bacteria except which of the following:
    a. they can only be seen with a microscope.
    c. they are one celled microorganisms.
    b. they can exist everywhere.
    d. they have both plant and animal characteristics. ____

23. Most bacteria are nonpathogenic which means they are harmless organisms that may perform _____ functions and are safe to come in contact with since they do not cause disease or harm.
    a. limited
    c. meaningless
    b. sporadic
    d. useful ____

24. A nonscientific term for disease-producing organisms is known as _____.
    a. parasite   c. germs
    b. toxin   d. virus   _____

25. Which type of cocci grow in clusters like a bunch of grapes?
    a. Streptococci   c. Staphylococci
    b. Bacilli   d. Diplococci   _____

26. Spherical bacteria that grow in pairs and causes diseases such as pneumonia are _____.
    a. staphylococci   c. streptococci
    b. bacilli   d. diplococci   _____

27. Spirilla bacteria are divided into two groups: Treponema papillida which causes syphilis and Borrelia burgdorferi which causes _____.
    a. Lyme disease   c. typhoid fever
    b. tetanus or lockjaw   d. chronic pneumonia   _____

28. Different bacteria move in different ways and self-movement is known as _____.
    a. migration   c. evolution
    b. motility   d. locomotion   _____

29. When bacteria reach their largest size, they divide into two new cells—a process called _____.
    a. mitosis   c. subdivision
    b. detachment   d. binary fission   _____

30. Certain fungi and bacteria coat themselves with wax outer shells that are able to withstand long periods of famine, _____, and unsuitable temperatures.
    a. moisture   c. warmth
    b. darkness   d. dryness   _____

31. Tissue inflammation creates a fluid known as _____.
    a. discharge   c. mucous
    b. pus   d. matter   _____

32. A main cause of infection from a salon's whirlpool foot spa can be traced to debris building up to create a thin coating called _____.
    a. biofilm   c. biocoat
    b. biogerm   d. biotissue   _____

33. When a disease spreads from one person to another, it is said to be _____.
   a. a spreading disease
   c. a transmittable disease
   b. an endemic disease
   d. a contagious disease   ____

34. Redness, heat, pain, and swelling are an indication of _____.
   a. an allergy
   c. contamination
   b. an inflammation
   d. contagion   ____

35. A parasitic submicroscopic particle that infects and resides in the cells of a biological organism is known as _____.
   a. an infection
   c. a virus
   b. a disease
   d. an inflammation   ____

36. Nail technicians may want to ask their doctor about getting vaccinated against _____.
   a. hepatitis A
   c. hepatitis C
   b. hepatitis B
   d. hepatitis D   ____

37. Hepatitis is a bloodborne disease that damages which part of the body?
   a. Heart
   c. Lungs
   b. Brain
   d. Liver   ____

38. A person can be infected with HIV for many years without having symptoms, but testing can determine if a person is infected within _____ months after exposure to the virus.
   a. one
   c. three
   b. two
   d. six   ____

39. Single-cell organisms that grow in irregular masses that include molds, mildews, and yeasts and can produce contagious diseases such as ringworm are called _____.
   a. fungi
   c. abscesses
   b. bacteria
   d. bacilli   ____

40. A(n) _____ is an organism that grows, feeds, and shelters on or in another organism without contributing anything to the other organism's survival.
   a. fungus
   c. parasite
   b. carrier
   d. host   ____

41. Immunity against disease can be either _____.
   a. natural or acquired
   c. basic or advanced
   b. simple or complex
   d. organic or inorganic   ____

42. When you remove all visible dirt and debris from something using soap and water, you _____ it.
    a. disinfect   c. clean
    b. sterilize   d. rinse   _____

43. What is the accepted method for testing an autoclave?
    a. Distillation test c. Acid test
    b. pH test   d. Spore test   _____

44. Disinfectants are appropriate on _____.
    a. soft surfaces   c. nonporous surfaces
    b. visibly dirty surfaces   d. porous surfaces   _____

45. Unless the label states otherwise, implements being disinfected must remain immersed in the disinfectant for at least _____ minutes.
    a. 3   c. 10
    b. 5   d. 15   _____

46. The technical term for quats is _____.
    a. quaternary ammonium   c. quaternary ammonium
       composites   compounds
    b. qualified ammonium   d. quaternary aluminum
       composites   composites   _____

47. Phenolic disinfectants are powerful tuberculocidal disinfectants that have a _____.
    a. very high pH   c. neutral pH
    b. very low pH   d. an acidic pH   _____

48. Household bleach, an effective disinfectant for salon uses,

    _____.
    a. is completely   c. is safe for the eyes
       noncorrosive
    b. can cause skin irritation   d. is safe for use on
                                      plastics   _____

49. When using disinfectants, you must always _____ and avoid skin and eye contact.
    a. wear gloves   c. estimate the amount
                             to mix
    b. pre-mix large amounts   d. place in an unmarked
                                  container   _____

50. A multiuse, or _____, item can be cleaned, disinfected, and used on more than one person, even if the item is accidentally exposed to blood or body fluid.
    a. disposable
    b. plastic
    c. porous
    d. reusable ____

51. If client packs are allowed in your state, each item must be properly cleaned, disinfected, and _____ before being placed in the pack.
    a. wiped
    b. rinsed
    c. dried
    d. polished ____

52. A nail technician's tools must be cleaned and disinfected _____.
    a. after each use
    b. at the end of the day
    c. at the end of the week
    d. when time permits ____

53. What types of cleaners are specially designed to break down stubborn films and residue of pedicure products from foot spas?
    a. Quats
    b. Chelating soaps
    c. Bleach
    d. Degreaser ____

54. Contact with nonintact skin, blood, bloody fluid, or other potentially infectious materials that results from the nail technician's performance is known as _____.
    a. blood event
    b. exposure accident
    c. exposure event
    d. exposure incident ____

55. Who publishes the Standard Precautions?
    a. The FDA
    b. The FBI
    c. The CDC
    d. The EPA ____

56. If there is an exposure incident, what is your next step after you stop the service and put on gloves?
    a. Apply pressure and clean the injury with an antiseptic.
    b. Clean and disinfect your entire workstation.
    c. Apply an adhesive bandage to completely cover the wound.
    d. Wash your hands with soap and water and discard contaminated objects. ____

57. When cleaning and disinfecting a whirlpool foot spa after a client, what is the next step after draining all the water from the basin?
    a. Put on gloves and safety glasses.
    b. Refill the basin with clean water to cover the jets.
    c. Rinse the basin with clean water and drain.
    d. Scrub all visible residue from inside the basin with soap and water. ____

CHAPTER 6: GENERAL ANATOMY AND PHYSIOLOGY

1. The study of the tiny structures found in tissue is called
   _____.
   a. anatomy
   b. histology
   c. physiology
   d. psychology
   ____

2. The cells of all living things are composed of a substance
   called _____.
   a. protoplasm
   b. cytoplasm
   c. nuclei
   d. membranes
   ____

3. Mitosis occurs when _____.
   a. the daughter cells are dissolved
   b. one cell splits into two identical cells
   c. two cells join to become one
   d. one cell splits into two cells
   ____

4. Unfavorable conditions that will inhibit a cell's growth and
   reproduction include all but which of the following?
   a. Excess toxins
   b. Lack of oxygen
   c. Restricted blood flow
   d. Adequate food
   ____

5. The process of building up larger molecules from smaller
   ones is called _____.
   a. metabolism
   b. anabolism
   c. catabolism
   d. botulism
   ____

6. Which type of tissue binds together, protects, and supports
   the various parts of the body?
   a. Epithelial tissue
   b. Liquid tissue
   c. Connective tissue
   d. Muscular tissue
   ____

7. Which type of tissue lines the respiratory organs?
   a. Epithelial tissue
   b. Nerve tissue
   c. Muscular tissue
   d. Liquid tissue
   ____

8. Which organ supplies oxygen to the blood?
   a. Brain
   b. Heart
   c. Liver
   d. Lungs
   ____

9. The _____ system purifies the body by eliminating
   waste matter.
   a. excretory
   b. circulatory
   c. lymphatic
   d. skeletal
   ____

10. The human skeleton eventually has _____ bones after some have fused together.
    a. 130
    b. 206
    c. 234
    d. 412
    _____

11. About one-third of bone is organic matter, and the other two-thirds are primarily composed of _____.
    a. phosphate compounds
    b. lead compounds
    c. minerals
    d. iron compounds
    _____

12. Which of the following is an example of an immovable joint?
    a. Skull
    b. Knees
    c. Hips
    d. Elbows
    _____

13. The _____ is the inner and larger bone of the forearm, attached to the wrist, and located on the side of the little finger.
    a. carpus
    b. metacarpus
    c. radius
    d. ulna
    _____

14. The phalanges are the bones of the _____.
    a. forearm and hand
    b. fingers and toes
    c. arm and fingers
    d. toes and feet
    _____

15. The _____, also called the accessory bone, forms the kneecap joint.
    a. patella
    b. fibula
    c. femur
    d. tibia
    _____

16. Which of the following is a tarsal bone?
    a. Tibia
    b. Navicular
    c. Fibula
    d. Femur
    _____

17. How many muscles are there in the human body?
    a. About 80
    b. More than 600
    c. Fewer than 200
    d. About 900
    _____

18. Which type of muscle tissue is found in the internal organs of the body, such as the digestive system?
    a. Striated muscle
    b. Cardiac muscle
    c. Nonstriated muscle
    d. Skeletal muscle
    _____

19. Which of the following is not one of the three parts of a muscle?
    a. Nucleus
    b. Origin
    c. Insertion
    d. Belly
    _____

20. Muscular tissue can be stimulated by massage which is pressure and friction created by hand, electric vibrator, or _____.
    a. moist heat
    b. electrical current
    c. nerve impulses
    d. water jets
    _____

21. Where is the latissimus dorsi located?
    a. The lower back
    b. The upper back
    c. The chest
    d. The abdomen
    _____

22. The _____ is the large muscle that covers the entire back of the upper arm and extends the forearm.
    a. deltoid
    b. tricep
    c. bicep
    d. pronator
    _____

23. The _____ are the muscles that separate the fingers.
    a. abductors
    b. adductors
    c. pronators
    d. extensors
    _____

24. The _____ originates at the upper portion of the fibula and bends the foot down.
    a. gastrocnemius
    b. tibialis anterior
    c. soleus
    d. peroneus longus
    _____

25. The _____ moves the lesser toes and helps maintain balance while walking.
    a. abductor hallucis
    b. flexor digitorum brevis
    c. extensor digitorum longus
    d. flexor digiti minimi
    _____

26. The scientific study of the structure, function, and pathology of the nervous system is known as _____.
    a. psychology
    b. neurology
    c. anatomy
    d. physiology
    _____

27. The principal components of the nervous system include all but which of the following?
    a. Brain
    b. Spinal cord
    c. Carpus
    d. Nerves
    _____

28. The spinal cord originates in the _____.
    a. brain
    b. spinal column
    c. vertebrae
    d. trunk
    _____

29. There are how many pairs of cranial nerves?
    a. 4
    b. 12
    c. 16
    d. 22
    _____

30. The treelike branches of nerve fibers extending from the nerve cell that carry impulses toward the cell and receive impulses from other nerve cells are called _____.
    a. dendrites
    b. axons
    c. neurons
    d. valves
    _____

31. Which type of nerves carries impulses from the sense organs to the brain?
    a. Motor
    b. Receptor
    c. Afferent
    d. Digital
    _____

32. The _____ nerve, with its branches, supplies the fingers.
    a. radial
    b. median
    c. ulnar
    d. digital
    _____

33. The _____ nerve extends from behind the knee to wind around the head of the fibula to the front of the leg, where it divides into two branches.
    a. deep peroneal
    b. anterior tibial
    c. common peroneal
    d. musculocutaneous
    _____

34. The sural nerve supplies impulses to the skin on the _____.
    a. shoulders and back
    b. foot and leg
    c. hands and arms
    d. neck and chest
    _____

35. The lymphatics are also known as _____.
    a. lymph spaces
    b. lymph nodes
    c. lymph cells
    d. lymph vessels
    _____

36. What is the primary function of lymph?
    a. To carry waste and impurities away from the cells
    b. To deliver oxygen and deliver nutrients to the cells
    c. To collect oxygen from the lungs and deliver it to the blood
    d. To initiate clotting when the skin is cut
    _____

37. About how much does a human heart weigh?
    a. 9 ounces
    b. 16 ounces
    c. 2 pounds
    d. 4 pounds
    _____

38. The chambers of the heart include _____.
    a. the atria and the vesicles
    b. the aorta and the ventricles
    c. the atria and the ventricles
    d. the aorta and the vesicles
    _____

39. When oxygen-rich blood returns to the heart, it enters the _____.
    a. right atrium
    b. left atrium
    c. right ventricle
    d. left ventricle
    _____

40. When blood leaves the heart to flow throughout the body, it exits from the _____.
    a. right atrium
    b. left atrium
    c. right ventricle
    d. left ventricle   _____

41. Compared to arteries, veins are located _____.
    a. farther from the outer skin surface
    b. closer to the outer skin surface
    c. the same distance from the outer skin surface
    d. very deep within the body   _____

42. Blood comprises about _____ of the body's total weight.
    a. 1/3
    b. 3/16
    c. 1/20
    d. 1/50   _____

43. Blood is _____.
    a. 98 percent water
    b. sweet
    c. sticky
    d alkaline   _____

44. Blood in the arteries is _____.
    a. bright red
    b. dark red
    c. blue
    d. purple   _____

45. What are leukocytes?
    a. Red blood cells
    b. White blood cells
    c. A type of hemoglobin
    d. A type of platelet   _____

46. Platelets are _____.
    a. responsible for destroying disease
    b. responsible for carrying food to cells
    c. larger than red blood cells
    d. smaller than red blood cells   _____

47. Blood helps to equalize the body's temperature; seals leaks found in injured blood vessels; carries water, oxygen, and food to all cells; carries away carbon dioxide and other waste products; and _____.
    a. helps to equalize the body's weight
    b. closes openings found in the epidermis
    c. works with the immune system to protect the body
    d. combines proteins and sugar to make platelets   _____

48. What is the most complex organ of the endocrine system?
    a. Pineal gland
    b. Pancreas
    c. Pituitary gland
    d. Thyroid gland   _____

49. The organ that eliminates waste containing perspiration is the
    _____.
    a. kidneys   c. lungs
    b. skin   d. liver   _____

50. If deprived of oxygen, a person will die in within _____.
    a. minutes   c. hours
    b. seconds   d. days   _____

CHAPTER 7: SKIN STRUCTURE, GROWTH, AND NUTRITION

1. A physician engaged in the science of treating the skin, its structures, functions, and diseases is known as
_____.
   a. a podiatrist
   b. a dermatologist
   c. an oncologist
   d. an endocrinologist ____

2. The _____ is the largest organ of the body.
   a. heart
   b. liver
   c. skin
   d. large intestine ____

3. The skin _____ is the thinnest of the body.
   a. on the cheeks
   b. around the eyelids
   c. on the scalp
   d. between the fingers ____

4. Which layer of the skin is thinnest?
   a. The epidermis
   b. The dermis
   c. The subcutaneous
   d. The corium ____

5. Which layer of the skin is known as the spiny layer?
   a. Stratum lucidum
   b. Stratum granulosum
   c. Stratum spinosum
   d. Stratum germinativum ____

6. The _____ has special column-shaped cells that produce melanocytes.
   a. stratum corneum
   b. stratum lucidum
   c. stratum granulosum
   d. stratum germinativum ____

7. The dermis is the underlying or inner layer of the skin, which is also called the derma, corium, or _____.
   a. lucidum
   b. stratus
   c. cutis
   d. medulla ____

8. The subcutaneous tissue is a fatty layer found below the dermis, which is also called _____ tissue.
   a. derma
   b. adipose
   c. corium
   d. cutis ____

9. What are the two layers of the dermis?
   a. Papillary and reticular
   b. Superficial and papillary
   c. Reticular and deeper
   d. Tactile and superficial ____

10. Lymph, the clear fluids of the body that resemble blood plasma but contains only water and other _____, bathe the skin cells, remove toxins, and have immune functions.
   a. red blood cells
   b. platelets
   c. white blood cells
   d. colorless substances ____

11. Sensory nerve fibers react to heat, cold, pressure, and _____.
    a. vibration   c. pain
    b. noise   d. sleep   _____

12. The color of the skin depends primarily on _____.
    a. melanin   c. keloids
    b. phenol   d. sebum   _____

13. Eumelanin is _____ in color.
    a. red to yellow   c. brown to black
    b. yellow to orange   d. blue to brown   _____

14. Daily use of a sunscreen with a sun protection factor of at least _____ is recommended.
    a. 50   c. 8
    b. 45   d. 15   _____

15. Collagen fibers are interwoven with _____, a protein base similar to collagen that forms elastic tissue.
    a. elastin   c. wheal
    b. sebum   d. melanocytes   _____

16. The sudoriferous glands are also known as _____ glands.
    a. sebaceous   c. oil
    b. sweat   d. lymph   _____

17. Normally, 1 to 2 _____ of liquids containing salts are eliminated daily through sweat pores in the skin.
    a. ounces   c. pints
    b. quarts   d. liters   _____

18. Sebaceous glands are not found on which part of the body?
    a. Face   c. Forearms
    b. Scalp   d. Palms   _____

19. A comedo is a hair follicle filled with _____.
    a. pus and lymph   c. keratin and sebum
    b. keratin and lymph   d. pus and sebum   _____

20. An excellent moisturizer and lubricant that replenishes skin lipids while softening and smoothing is known as _____.
    a. squalene   c. lanolin
    b. glycerin   d. allantoin   _____

21. Sebum is secreted by the _____ glands and lubricates the skin, keeping it soft and pliable.
    a. sudoriferous
    c. secretory
    b. sebaceous
    d. pituitary
    _____

22. Water composes approximately _____ of body weight.
    a. 40 percent
    c. 60 percent
    b. 50 percent
    d. 70 percent
    _____

23. The amount of water needed by an individual varies, depending on _____ and the level of daily physical activity.
    a. age
    c. overall health
    b. body height
    d. body weight
    _____

24. It is recommended that men in general should drink _____ cups of water daily.
    a. 8
    c. 11
    b. 10
    d. 12
    _____

25. Which of the following has the greatest negative impact on how our skin ages?
    a. Health habits
    c. General lifestyle
    b. Sun exposure
    d. Disease
    _____

26. _____ energy contributes to the body's synthesis of vitamin D and other important minerals.
    a. UVB
    c. UVA
    b. Solar
    d. Artificial
    _____

27. UVA energy is deeper penetrating than _____ and causes the skin to tan by affecting the skin pigment.
    a. invisible light
    c. visible light
    b. solar light
    d. artificial light
    _____

28. For the best protection when UV exposure is the highest, an individual should avoid prolonged exposure to the sun during peak hours, which usually occurs between
    _____.
    a. 8:00 a.m. and 10:00 a.m.
    c. 3:00 p.m. and 4:00 p.m.
    b. 10:00 a.m. and 3:00 p.m.
    d. 4:00 p.m. and 5:00 p.m.
    _____

29. A protein similar to collagen that forms elastic tissue is known as _____.
    a. keratin
    c. eumelanin
    b. melanin
    d. elastin
    _____

30. Which of the following people are *most* susceptible to sun damage?
    a. Redheads and brunettes
    b. Redheads and blue-eyed blondes
    c. Blue-eyed and brown-eyed brunettes
    d. Blue-eyed and green-eyed brunettes

    _____

31. Changes in the size, shape, or coloration of a mole are cause _____.
    a. to have it removed
    b. to monitor it closely
    c. to apply moisturizer
    d. to see a physician

    _____

32. Inhaling nicotine in tobacco causes the _____ and weakening of blood vessels that supply blood to the skin tissues.
    a. dilation
    b. thickening
    c. contraction
    d. expansion

    _____

33. A condition caused by heavy or excessive intake of alcohol, tobacco use, sun exposure, or other environmental factors is known as _____.
    a. telangiectasias
    b. eczema
    c. rosacea
    d. acne

    _____

34. Which type of lesions are nail technicians concerned with?
    a. Primary and tertiary
    b. Tertiary and secondary
    c. Primary and secondary
    d. Primary, secondary, and tertiary

    _____

35. A _____ is a large blister containing a watery fluid.
    a. cyst
    b. bulla
    c. papule
    d. macule

    _____

36. A spot or discoloration on the skin, such as a freckle, is known as _____.
    a. cyst
    b. vesicle
    c. tumor
    d. macule

    _____

37. An inflamed pimple containing pus is called a _____.
    a. pustule
    b. tubercle
    c. vesicle
    d. cyst

    _____

38. A thick scar resulting from excessive growth of fibrous tissue is called _____.
    a. a scale
    b. a crust
    c. a keloid
    d. an excoriation

    _____

39. A collection of blood trapped underneath the nail is called
    _____.
    a. a hematoma   c   an ulcer
    b. a cicatrix   d. a fissure   _____

40. Which of the following terms refers to a deficiency in
    perspiration?
    a. Miliaria rubra   c. Hyperhidrosis
    b. Anhidrosis   d. Bromhidrosis   _____

41. What is the least severe and most common type of skin
    cancer?
    a. Basal cell carcinoma   c. Malignant melanoma
    b. Squamous cell carcinoma   d. Benign melanoma   _____

42. Prolonged or repeated contact with many _____ will
    strip away skin oils, leaving the skin dry or damaged.
    a. solutions   c. solvents
    b. creams   d. antiseptics   _____

43. To avoid allergies when working with monomer liquids or
    UV gels, you should never _____ your own product
    blends.
    a. use   c. smooth
    b. touch   d. mix   _____

44. The _____ prevents absorption of a very large majority
    of what comes in contact with the surface of the skin,
    including cosmetic ingredients.
    a. dermis   c. sweat glands
    c. epidermis   d. cutis   _____

45. A substance that is needed for proper repair of the skin
    and various tissues, which also speeds up the healing
    processes of the body, is _____.
    a. vitamin C   c. vitamin D
    b. vitamin A   d. vitamin E   _____

CHAPTER 8: NAIL STRUCTURE AND GROWTH

1. The hard protective plate located at the end of the finger or toe is called the _____.
   a. natural nail
   b. cuticle
   c. matrix
   d. ligament
   _____

2. The fingernails and toenails are part of which body system?
   a. Digestive system
   b. Integumentary system
   c. Reproductive system
   d. Respiratory system
   _____

3. The _____ of the nails can reflect the general health of the body.
   a. length
   b. thickness
   c. width
   d. overall appearance
   _____

4. Which of the following is technically referred to as the onyx?
   a. The matrix
   b. The natural nail
   c. The eponychium
   d. The bed epithelium
   _____

5. The natural nail is primarily composed of what substance?
   a. Bile
   b. Hyponychium
   c. Keratin
   d. Carbohydrates
   _____

6. A normal, healthy nail is firm and flexible, shiny, slightly pink in color with a _____ surface.
   a. smooth
   b. brittle
   c. hardened
   d. thin
   _____

7. The keratin in natural nails is _____ the keratin in hair or skin.
   a. the same as
   b. darker than
   c. softer than
   d. more durable than
   _____

8. The nail plate is relatively _____ to water, allowing it to pass much more easily than it will pass through normal skin of equal thickness.
   a. resistant
   b. opposed
   c. porous
   d. absorbent
   _____

9. The lower the water content in the nail, the _____ the nail becomes.
   a. more rigid
   b. less rigid
   c. darker
   d. lighter
   _____

10. The portion of living skin that supports the nail plate as it grows toward the free edge is called the _____.
   a. nail groove
   c. nail fold
   b. nail unit
   d. nail bed   _____

11. The area under the nail plate has a _____ appearance extending from the lunula to just before the free edge of the nail.
   a. bluish
   c. greenish
   b. pinkish
   d. yellowish   _____

12. Where are the nail plate cells formed?
   a. The bed epithelium
   c. The matrix
   b. The bone marrow
   d. The ligaments   _____

13. What is the whitish half-moon shape at the base of the nail called?
   a. The nail plate
   c. The eponychium
   b. The lunula
   d. The hyponychium   _____

14. The matrix area contains nerves, lymph, and _____ to nourish the matrix cells.
   a. water supply
   c. blood vessels
   b. plasma
   d. arteries   _____

15. The _____ is the most visible and functional part of the nail unit.
   a. cuticle
   c. nail plate
   b. bed epithelium
   d. matrix   _____

16. The free edge _____.
   a. is an integral part of the matrix
   c. attaches directly to the nail bed
   b. extends over the tip of the finger or toe
   d. guides the nail plate along the nail bed   _____

17. The cuticle is the dead, _____ tissue attached to the nail plate.
   a. colorless
   c. pinkish
   b. flaky
   d. hardened   _____

18. Cuticle tissue is incredibly _____ and difficult to remove from the nail plate.
   a. easy
   c. difficult
   b. tricky
   d. tedious   _____

19. The living skin at the base of the nail plate covering the matrix area is the _____.
   a. eponychium
   b. hyponychium
   c. cuticle
   d. matrix
   _____

20. The _____ is the slightly thickened layer of skin that lies between the fingertip and the free edge of the nail plate.
   a. eponychium
   b. hyponychium
   c. cuticle
   d. matrix
   _____

21. A tough band of fibrous tissue that connects bones or holds an organ in place is called _____.
   a. a tendon
   b. a tibia
   c. a group
   d. a ligament
   _____

22. Nail technicians are allowed to gently push back the eponychium but are prohibited from cutting or trimming any part of the eponychium because it is _____.
   a. a vital part of the nail unit
   b. necessary for nail shape
   c. critical to nail health
   d. living skin
   _____

23. Cuticle conditioners are designed for the eponychium, lateral sidewalls, and _____.
   a. cuticle
   b. nail plate
   c. finger tips
   d. hyponychium
   _____

24. Cuticle removers, when carefully applied to the nail plate, can speed removal of stubborn _____.
   a. sidewall tissue
   b. nail bed tissue
   c. free edge tissue
   d. cuticle tissue
   _____

25. Ligaments are located at the base of the _____ and around the edges of the nail bed.
   a. nail plate
   b. matrix
   c. sidewalls
   d. lunula
   _____

26. The _____ are folds of normal skin that surround the nail plate.
   a. nail folds
   b. nail grooves
   c. nail beds
   d. matrices
   _____

27. The sidewall, also called the _____, is the fold of skin overlapping the side of the nail.
   a. vertical nail fold
   b. corrugation
   c. horizontal nail fold
   d. lateral nail fold
   _____

28. A normal nail grows forward from the _____ and extends over the tip of the finger.
    a. matrix
    b. free edge
    c. lunula
    d. nail bed
    _____

29. The length, width, and curvature of the _____ determine the thickness, width, and curvature of the natural nail plate.
    a. ligament
    b. bed epithelium
    c. matrix
    d. free edge
    _____

30. What can be done to make the nail plate grow thicker?
    a. Basic manicures
    b. Nothing
    c. Hot oil manicures
    d. Spa manicures
    _____

31. Nails grow slowest at what time of year?
    a. Summer
    b. Spring
    c. Fall
    d. Winter
    _____

32. The nail of the _____ grows fastest.
    a. thumb
    b. index finger
    c. middle finger
    d. pinkie finger
    _____

33. Nails of _____ grow at a slower rate than others.
    a. children
    b. adults
    c. adolescents
    d. the elderly
    _____

34. Because of hormonal changes in the body, nail growth, _____ during the last trimester of pregnancy.
    a. increases dramatically
    b. decreases dramatically
    c. stops altogether
    d. varies dramatically
    _____

35. What causes the dramatic increases and decreases in the rate of nail growth during and after pregnancy?
    a. A lack of prenatal vitamins
    b. The use of prenatal vitamins
    c. Changes in diet
    d. Hormonal changes
    _____

36. Compared to the matrix found on fingernails, the matrix found on toenails is _____.
    a. shorter
    b. longer
    c. darker in color
    d. lighter in color
    _____

37. Compared to fingernails, toenails grow _____.
    a. thinner
    b. softer
    c. slower
    d. faster
    _____

38. How long does the replacement of the natural fingernail take?
   a. 2–3 weeks
   c. 2–4 months
   b. 6–8 weeks
   d. 4–6 months   _____

39. How long does it take for the natural replacement of
   a toenail?
   a. 8–10 weeks
   c. 9–12 months
   b. 4–6 months
   d. 12–16 months   _____

40. The natural nail is considered an appendage of the
   _____.
   a. skin
   c. hair
   b. bone
   d. nail bed   _____

41. The surface of a normal, healthy nail _____.
   a. has hollows
   c. is unspotted
   b. has wavy ridges
   d. has excessive
      curvature   _____

42. Oil-based nail conditioners _____.
   a. are not recommended
   b. can improve nail
      flexibility
   c. can increase water loss
   d. can soften cuticles   _____

43. Nail folds form the nail groove or _____ on each
   side of the nail.
   a. furrow
   c. trench
   b. depression
   d. wrinkle   _____

44. As a person ages, parts of the nail matrix begin to
   permanently slow down production, causing the plate
   to develop a series of _____ running the length
   of the plate.
   a. wavy ridges
   c. wavy furrows
   b. hard depressions
   d. narrow grooves   _____

CHAPTER 9: NAIL DISORDERS AND DISEASES

1. A normal healthy nail is shiny and slightly pink in color, with more _____ tones in some races.
   - a. light green
   - b. light brown
   - c. beige/yellow
   - d. blue/green
   _____

2. It is likely that _____ of your clients have experienced one or more types of common nail disorders.
   - a. none
   - b. most
   - c. very few
   - d. about half
   _____

3. A nail disorder is a condition caused by injury or _____.
   - a. genetics
   - b. over buffing
   - c. disease
   - d. nipping
   _____

4. Bruised nails are characterized by a blood clot that forms under the plate, forming a _____ spot.
   - a. dark purplish
   - b. light pinkish
   - c. dull greenish
   - d. bright bluish
   _____

5. Nail ridges, which are actually grooves, grow in which direction?
   - a. Any directions
   - b. Horizontally
   - c. Diagonally
   - d. Vertically
   _____

6. Ridges are _____.
   - a. normal in younger clients
   - b. normal in older clients
   - c. a sign of poor nutrition
   - d. a sign of poor health
   _____

7. Eggshell nails are noticeably thin, white nail plates that are _____ than normal nails.
   - a. much more flexible
   - b. much firmer
   - c. much less flexible
   - d. much more rigid
   _____

8. When working on eggshell nails, it is recommended that you use an abrasive board with a grit of _____.
   - a. 80 or lower
   - b. 120 or higher
   - c. 240 or higher
   - d. 80–120
   _____

9. Which way do Beau's lines typically run on the nail plate?
   - a. Vertically
   - b. Horizontally
   - c. Diagonally
   - d. Any direction
   _____

10. Beau's lines occur because the matrix _____ producing nail cells for several weeks or months.
   - a. speeds up in
   - b. has interruptions in
   - c. totally stops
   - d. slows down in
   _____

11. Which of these conditions is characterized by the living skin around the nail plate splitting and tearing?
    a. Hangnail
    c. Nail pterygium
    b. Onychophagy
    d. Pincer nail
    _____

12. Signs of an infection of the nails are redness, pain, swelling, or _____.
    a. bruising
    c. bleeding
    b. pus
    d. splitting
    _____

13. What color are leukonychia spots?
    a. Purple
    c. Blue
    b. Yellow
    d. White
    _____

14. Leukonychia spots result from _____.
    a. a vitamin deficiency
    c. damage to the matrix
    b. a calcium deficiency
    d. a zinc deficiency
    _____

15. Melanonychia presents as a _____ of the nails.
    a. cracking
    c. lightening
    b. splitting
    d. darkening
    _____

16. Melanonychia is a fairly common occurrence and considered normal in _____, but could be indicative of a disease condition in Caucasians.
    a. African Americans or Asians
    c. Italians and Asians
    b. Hispanics and African Americans
    d. Greeks and Asians
    _____

17. Which of these conditions is caused by nail biting?
    a. Onychocryptosis
    c. Onychia
    b. Onychophagy
    d. Onychomadesis
    _____

18. The technical term for split or brittle nails with a series of lengthwise ridges is _____.
    a. plicatured nail
    c. nail pterygium
    b. splinter hemorrhages
    d. onychorrhexis
    _____

19. How often should a client with onychorrhexis use a high-quality, penetrating nail oil?
    a. Once daily
    c. Twice daily
    b. Once weekly
    d. Twice weekly
    _____

20. The condition known as plicatured nail often leads to _____ nails.
    a. ingrown
    c. split
    b. bruised
    d. brittle
    _____

21. Skin is stretched by the nail plate in clients with _____.
   a. pincer nail   c. nail psoriasis
   b. trumpet nail   d. nail pterygium   ____

22. What should you do if a client has a typical case of pincer nail?
   a. Refer her to a physician.   c. Aggressively file and shape the nail.
   b. Carefully trim and file the nail.   d. Apply ridge filler and nail polish.   ____

23. Fungi are _____.
   a. parasites   c. germs
   b. bacteria   d. mold   ____

24. Nail fungi are of concern to the nail salon because they are contagious and can be transmitted through _____.
   a. personal touch   c. dry air
   b. contaminated implements   d. cleansing antiseptics   ____

25. A typical bacterial infection on the nail plate can be identified in the early stages as a _____ spot.
   a. blue-green   c. red-purple
   b. yellow-green   d. brown-black   ____

26. Which of the following colors indicates the most advanced nail infection?
   a. Yellow   c. Brown
   b. Green   d. Black   ____

27. A form of dramatically increased nail curvature is called _____.
   a. bugle nails   c. trumpet nails
   b. horned nails   d. plicatured nails   ____

28. Which of these conditions presents as an inflammation of the nail matrix followed by shedding of the natural nail plate?
   a. Onychia   c. Onychocryptosis
   b. Onychosis   d. Onycholysis   ____

29. The technical term for ingrown nails is _____.
   a. paronychia   c. onychocryptosis
   b. onychomadesis   d. onychomycosis   ____

30. The technical term for separation and failing off of a nail from the nail bed is _____.
   a. paronychia   c. onychocryptosis
   b. onychomadesis   d. onychomycosis   ____

31. Which of the following does not usually cause onycholysis?
    a. Illness
    b. Physical injury
    c. Allergic reactions
    d. Trauma _____

32. Onychomadesis can be traced to a localized infection, _____, or a severe systemic illness.
    a. injury to the free edge
    b. injury to the cuticle
    c. injury to the matrix
    d. injury to the lunula _____

33. What effect does nail psoriasis have on the nails?
    a. Splitting
    b. Pitting
    c. Crumbling
    d. Darkening _____

34. Nail psoriasis can cause yellowish to reddish spots underneath the nail plate, called _____.
    a. port blotches
    b. leukonychia spots
    c. bleach blots
    d. salmon patches _____

35. Paronychia is _____.
    a. a bacterial inflammation of the tissues surrounding the nail
    b. the separation and falling off of a nail from the nail bed
    c. red itchy patches of skin between the toes
    d. depressions running across the width of the nail plate _____

36. Which of the following people is likely to be most prone to paronychia?
    a. A carpenter
    b. A nurse
    c. An electrician
    d. An attorney _____

37. Nail psoriasis can cause the surface of the plate to look like it has been filed with a coarse abrasive or may _____.
    a. create a ragged free edge
    b. create white spots
    c. create a hangnail
    d. a damaged lunula _____

38. Which of the following conditions is a severe inflammation of the nail in which a lump of red tissue grows up from the nail bed to the nail plate?
    a. Melanonychia
    b. Nail pterygium
    c. Pyogenic granuloma
    d. Onychorrhexis _____

39. What is the medical term for red itchy patches of skin on the bottom of the feet?
    a. Tinea capitis
    b. Tinea pedis
    c. Tinea versicolor
    d. Tinea cruris _____

40. A fungal infection of the feet is *most* likely to strike between the _____ toes.
    a. first and second
    b. second and third
    c. third and fourth
    d. fourth and fifth ____

41. If a client has a fungal infection on the foot, you should recommend _____.
    a. changing wool socks twice daily
    b. changing shoes at least twice daily
    c. changing white cotton socks twice daily
    d. placing cotton with antiseptic between the toes ____

42. Which of these terms refers to a fungal infection of the nail plate?
    a. Onychomycosis
    b. Onychocryptosis
    c. Onychomadesis
    d. Pyogenic granuloma ____

43. What causes ridges?
    a. Physical injury
    b. Uneven nail growth
    c. Certain medications
    d. Certain illnesses ____

44. Plicatured nail figuratively means _____.
    a. brittle nail
    b. cracked nail
    c. spiraled nail
    d. folded nail ____

45. Nail pterygium is an abnormal condition that occurs when skin is _____ the nail plate.
    a. softened around
    b. hardened at the edge of
    c. stretched by
    d. detached from ____

CHAPTER 10: THE BASICS OF CHEMISTRY

1. Which branch of science focuses on the study of substances that contain the element carbon?
   - a. Inorganic chemistry
   - b. Chemistry
   - c. Organic chemistry
   - d. Geology _____

2. All living things, or things that were once alive, contain _____.
   - a. oxygen
   - b. carbon
   - c. hydrogen
   - d. nitrogen _____

3. Which of the following is not an organic substance?
   - a. Air
   - b. Poison ivy
   - c. Motor oil
   - d. Nail enhancements _____

4. The study of substances that do not contain carbon but may contain hydrogen is _____.
   - a. biology
   - b. organic chemistry
   - c. inorganic chemistry
   - d. geology _____

5. Matter is any substance that occupies space and has _____ or weight.
   - a. shape
   - b. texture
   - c. size
   - d. mass _____

6. Which of the following is not a chemical?
   - a. Light
   - b. Granite
   - c. Water
   - d. Sand _____

7. Energy _____.
   - a. occupies space
   - b. has mass
   - c. has chemical properties
   - d. is not matter _____

8. What is the letter symbol for carbon?
   - a. cn
   - b. C
   - c. Ca
   - d. ca _____

9. The smallest chemical particle of an element that retains the properties of that element is _____.
   - a. an atom
   - b. a molecule
   - c. a cell
   - d. a nucleus _____

10. What is the symbol for atmospheric oxygen?
    - a. O
    - b. O_2
    - c. O_3
    - d. CO_2. _____

11. How many atoms are in a molecule?
    a. None
    b. Only one
    c. Two or more
    d. No more than two   _____

12. Millions of chemical reactions occur in the body
    every _____, which is what keeps us alive.
    a. day
    b. hour
    c. minute
    d. second   _____

13. Common table salt is an example of _____.
    a. a compound element
    b. a common atom
    c. a compound molecule
    d. an emulsion   _____

14. When water boils it _____.
    a. changes its physical form to a gas
    b. changes its physical form to a liquid
    c. is no longer H_2O
    d. undergoes a chemical change   _____

15. Which of the following has a definite volume, but not a definite
    shape?
    a. Solids
    b. Liquids
    c. Gases
    d. Vapors   _____

16. Weight is an example of _____.
    a. a physical property
    b. a chemical property
    c. a substantive property
    d. a solid property   _____

17. When an abrasive file is used on the nail plate and both
    the nail plate and file are changed, _____ occurs.
    a. a chemical reaction
    b. an endothermic reaction
    c. a chemical change
    d. a physical change   _____

18. All atoms, elements, elemental molecules, and _____
    are pure substances.
    a. matter
    b. compound molecules
    c. liquids
    d. compound atoms   _____

19. Salt water is an example of _____.
    a. an emulsion
    b. a suspension
    c. a physical mixture
    d. a pure substance   _____

20. A _____ is a stable, uniform blend of two or more
    substances.
    a. solute
    b. solution
    c. solvent
    d. suspension   _____

21. Water and oil are _____.
    a. immiscible liquids   c. mutually soluble
    b. miscible liquids   d. easily mixed   ____

22. All matter exists in one of five different physical forms, including solid, liquid, gas, vapor, and _____.
    a. lymph   c. blood
    b. milk   d. plasma   ____

23. The binding agent that allows immiscible liquids to join together in an emulsion is called _____.
    a. a conjoiner   c. a solvent
    b. an emulsifier   d. an ion   ____

24. A properly formulated emulsion, stored under ideal conditions, can be stable for up to _____.
    a. 6 months   c. 3 years
    b. 1 year   d. 10 years   ____

25. The tail of a surfactant molecule is _____.
    a. hydrophilic   c. exothermic
    b. lipophilic   d. endothermic   ____

26. Mayonnaise is an example of _____.
    a. an oil-in-water emulsion c. a solution
    b. a water-in-oil emulsion d. a suspension   ____

27. Foot balm is an example of _____.
    a. an oil-in-water emulsion c. a solution
    b. a water-in-oil emulsion d. a suspension   ____

28. Pomades and pastes are made with a combination of petrolatum and what two other substances?
    a. Calcium and talc   c. Oil and wax
    b. Oil and talc   d. Wax and calcium   ____

29. Volatile alcohol is alcohol that _____.
    a. evaporates easily
    b. does not evaporate easily
    c. is flammable
    d. is inflammable   ____

30. Glycerin is _____ substance.
    a. a bitter   c. an oily
    b. a brown   d. a colorful   ____

31. A volatile organic compound contains which of the following?
    a. Nitrogen   c. Silicon
    b. Talc   d. Carbon   _____

32. An atom or molecule that carries an unbalanced electrical
    charge is called _____.
    a. an anion   c. a cation
    b. an ion   d. an electron   _____

33. When ionization occurs, the resulting ions _____.
    a. have opposite electrical charges
    b. have the same electrical charges
    c. have no electrical charge
    d. a negative electrical charge   _____

34. The more _____ ions a substance has, the more acidic
    it will be.
    a. carbon   c. hydroxide
    b. nitrogen   d. hydrogen   _____

35. A product must contain _____ to have a pH.
    a. silicon   c. water
    b. oxygen   d. alcohol   _____

36. Pure water has a _____ pH.
    a. neutral   c. alkaline
    b. acidic   d. ionized   _____

37. A solution is neutral if its pH is _____.
    a. 0.0   c. 7.0
    b. 1.0   d. 10.0   _____

38. The pH scale ranges from _____.
    a. 1–10   c. 1–14
    b. 0–14   d. 0–10   _____

39. A pH of 8 is _____ than a pH of 7.
    a. 100 times more acidic   c. 20 times more alkaline
    b. 10 times more alkaline   d. 100 times more alkaline   _____

40. An acidic solution will turn litmus paper from _____.
    a. white to black   c. red to blue
    b. black to white   d. blue to red   _____

41. An alkali _____.
    a. has a pH less than 7.0
    b. has a pH more than 7.0
    c. turn litmus paper from blue to red
    d. is safe in the eyes   ____

42. Nail polish is an example of _____.
    a. an inorganic substance   c. a volatile compound
    b. an organic substance   d. a solution   ____

43. Electricity is considered to be _____.
    a. matter   c. a chemical
    b. energy   d. a mineral   ____

44. How many naturally occurring elements are there?
    a. 67   c. 109
    b. 90   d. 117   ____

45. A special type of ingredient used in nail polish dryers and skin
    protectants is _____.
    a. alcohol   c. silicone
    b. glycerin   d. antiseptic   ____

CHAPTER 11: NAIL PRODUCT CHEMISTRY SIMPLIFIED

1. Which of the following is not a chemical?
   - a. Light
   - b. Water
   - c. Soil
   - d. Oxygen   _____

2. Petroleum oil can be chemically converted into _____.
   - a. sugar
   - b. water
   - c. acetone
   - d. vitamin C   _____

3. In medieval times, alchemists searched in vain for ways to turn _____ into _____.
   - a. water; wine
   - b. wine; water
   - c. gold; lead
   - d. lead; gold   _____

4. Vapors are formed when liquids _____ into the air.
   - a. spray
   - b. lift
   - c. boil
   - d. evaporate   _____

5. Which of the following are a blend of soot-like particles mixed with vapors?
   - a. Fumes
   - b. Gases
   - c. Solvents
   - d. Emulsions   _____

6. A chemical that causes two surfaces to stick together is _____.
   - a. a plasticizer
   - b. an adhesive
   - c. a monomer
   - d. a polymer   _____

7. A nail polish base coat is a type of _____.
   - a. wrap
   - b. oligomer
   - c. primer
   - d. initiator   _____

8. Which of the following is not a basic type of primer?
   - a. Acid-based
   - b. Nonacid
   - c. Acid-free
   - d. Dual acid   _____

9. A substance that can cause visible and possibly permanent skin or eye damage is _____.
   - a. a corrosive
   - b. an adhesive
   - c. a polymer
   - d. a catalyst   _____

10. A corrosive acid-based primer can cause painful burns and _____ to soft tissue and eyes.
    - a. cuts
    - b. nicks
    - c. scars
    - d. scalds   _____

11. How much primer is typically recommended for most clients?
    a. None
    c. 2–3 coats
    b. 1 coat
    d. Up to 10 coats _____

12. Which type of primer contains methacrylic acid?
    a. Acid-base primer
    c. Nonacid primer
    b. Dual-acid primer
    d. Acid-free primer _____

13. Scrubbing the nail plate gets rid of the bacteria and
    _____ that cause fingernail infections.
    a. mold
    c. mildew
    b. debris
    d. fungi _____

14. The effects of a nail dehydrator will typically wear off
    within _____ minutes.
    a. 15
    c. 45
    b. 30
    d. 60 _____

15. An abrasive or buffer of _____ grit is recommended
    for preparing the nail plate for a nail enhancement product.
    a. 80
    c. 240
    b. 160
    d. 400 _____

16. The thinner the nail plate, the _____ it will be.
    a. weaker
    c. wider
    b. stronger
    d. longer _____

17. Ideally, the nail plate should be _____ before you
    apply a nail enhancement product.
    a. thick and weak
    c. thick and strong
    b. thin and weak
    d. thin and strong _____

18. _____ filing damages both the nail plate and the
    underlying sensitive tissues of the nail bed.
    a. Routine
    c. Strong
    b. Natural
    d. Rough _____

19. Overfiling the nail can lead to free-edge product separation,
    which is also known as _____.
    a. curling
    c. chipping
    b. splintering
    d. speckling _____

20. Proper preparation of the nail plate for nail enhancements
    includes removing all dead tissue for the side walls and
    _____ as well as bacteria, fungi, oil, and moisture from
    the nail plate.
    a. eponychium
    c. nail bed
    b. cuticle
    d. free edge _____

21. Soaking the nail plate in any liquid, including water and acetone, will temporarily soften the nail plate's surface for up to _____ minutes.
   a. 10   c. 30
   b. 20   d. 60   ____

22. If a coating cures or polymerizes, it undergoes a _____ reaction.
   a. hydrophilic   c. chemical
   b. lipophilic   d. physical   ____

23. The gigantic chains of molecules that make up UV gels, wraps, and adhesives are called _____.
   a. monomers   c. acrylates
   b. polymers   d. oligomers   ____

24. Polymers usually take which form?
   a. Solid   c. Gas
   b. Liquid   d. Vapor   ____

25. The terms cure, curing, or _____ are sometimes used synonymously with polymerization.
   a. softening   c. strengthening
   b. supporting   d. hardening   ____

26. Because nail plates are made of a protein called _____, they are considered polymers.
   a. melanin   c. keratin
   b. corpuscle   d. neuron   ____

27. The individual molecules that make up polymers are called _____.
   a. oligomers   c. UV stabilizers
   b. monomers   d. plasticizers   ____

28. What special ingredient triggers polymerization?
   a. The catalyst   c. The oligomer
   b. The initiator   d. The pigment   ____

29. How long does it take the polymer chains in nail enhancements to reach their ultimate lengths?
   a. Several days   c. Several seconds
   b. Several hours   d. Several minutes   ____

30. If a catalyst is added to a chemical reaction, what does it do?
   a. Nothing   c. Slows the reaction
   b. Stops the reaction   d. Speeds up the reaction   ____

31. Without _____, it would take UV gel products 2 or 3 hours to harden into nail enhancements.
    a. oligomers
    b. methyl methacrylate monomer (MMA)
    c. overexposure
    d. a cross-linker   _____

32. Liquid and powder systems use _____ that gather energy from the heat of the room or hand, while UV curing products use photoinitiators that derive their extra energy from exposure to UV.
    a. endothermic initiators   c. thermal initiators
    b. exothermic processors   d. photoprocessors   _____

33. Products with simple polymer chains are easily damaged by sharp impacts or _____.
    a. foods   c. marker inks
    b. solvents   d. heavy stresses   _____

34. Compared to uncross-linked products, cross-linked nail enhancements _____.
    a. take less time to remove in acetone
    b. take more time to remove in acetone
    c. take an equal amount of time to remove in acetone
    d. cannot be removed in acetone   _____

35. All nail enhancements and adhesives are based on a family of chemical ingredients called _____.
    a. polymers   c. acrylics
    b. monomers   d. coatings   _____

36. All monomer liquids and polymer powders are based on _____.
    a. acrylates   c. ambacrylates
    b. cyanoacrylates   d. methacrylates   _____

37. One of the reasons methyl methacrylate monomer (MMA) should not be used is because _____.
    a. it is extremely difficult to remove and will not dissolve in product removers
    b. it is a safe substance that is widely used for many applications
    c. it is not dangerous to inhale when there is proper ventilation
    d. it is not absorbed into the blood to affect health   _____

38. The vast majority of chemicals people come in contact with during a lifetime are completely safe and most are

_____.

a. beneficial   c. harmless
b. easy to use   d. nontoxic   ____

39. The majority of ingredients in evaporation coatings are _____ or quickly evaporating solvents.

a. highly flammable   c. volatile
b. polymer-based   d. monomer-based   ____

40. In nail enhancements, what is the function of a UV stabilizer?

a. To improve flexibility
b. To control color stability
c. To increase rigidity
d. To prevent chipping   ____

41. Which types of nail enhancements are made from organic substances?

a. All of them   c. Polymer-based
                          enhancements
b. None of them   d. Evaporation coatings ____

42. When problems with nail enhancements occur, they are least likely to be caused by _____.

a. improper maintenance c. improper removal
b. improper application d. nail products   ____

43. _____ said, "All substances are poisons; there is none that is not a poison. Only the dose differentiates between a poison and a remedy."

a. Jeff Pink   c. Paracelsus
b. Charles Revson   d. Queen Nefertiti   ____

44. Which of these statements about toxicity is true?

a. There are many substances that are completely nontoxic.
b. Toxicity is determined by overexposure.
c. No toxic product can be used safely.
d. Toxic products should never be used in the salon. ____

45. Local _____ systems are very effective ventilators and will help prevent overexposure if the manufacturer's recommendations are followed.

a. dust capture   c. air purifier
b. air cleanser   d. source capture   ____

CHAPTER 12: THE BASICS OF ELECTRICITY

1. The movement of particles around an atom that creates pure energy is called _____.
   a. lightning
   b. energetic flow
   c. electricity
   d. electron flow

   _____

2. Any substance that easily allows the flow of electricity with little resistance is known as _____.
   a. regulator
   b. insulator
   c. distractor
   d. conductor

   _____

3. The flow of electricity in a complete electric circuit is called _____.
   a. an electric current
   b. an electrical circuit
   c. a grounded circuit
   d. an energetic current

   _____

4. Electricity is a _____.
   a. form of light
   b. form of energy
   c. type of element
   d. type of molecule

   _____

5. A substance that does not easily transmit electricity is called _____.
   a. a conductor
   b. an insulator
   c. a rectifier
   d. a converter

   _____

6. Rubber, silk, _____, glass, and cement are all good insulators.
   a. copper
   b. wiring
   c. water
   d. wood

   _____

7. Pure water is a _____.
   a. good conductor
   b. poor conductor
   c. good insulator
   d. poor insulator

   _____

8. Insulators are also known as _____.
   a. chargers
   b. relays
   c. nonconductors
   d. transmitters

   _____

9. A complete electrical current is _____ that conducts electricity and provides a return path for the current.
   a. an open loop
   b. an open ring
   c. a figure eight
   d. a closed loop

   _____

10. The path of an electric current from the generating source through conductors and back to its original source is called _____ electrical circuit.
   a. a complete   c. a rectified
   b. an oscillating   d. a converted   _____

11. Constant, even-flowing current that travels in one direction only is commonly known as _____ current.
   a. an indirect   c. an alternating
   b. a direct   d. a uniform   _____

12. Rapid and interrupted current, flowing first in one direction and then in the opposite direction is commonly known as _____ current.
   a. an indirect   c. an alternating
   b. a direct   d. a uniform   _____

13. A cell phone uses _____ current.
   a. an indirect   c. an alternating
   b. a uniform   d. a direct   _____

14. Paraffin heaters use _____ current.
   a. a direct   c. an indirect
   b. an alternating   d. a uniform   _____

15. If you wanted to convert AC current to DC current, you would need to use _____.
   a. a rectifier   c. an insulator
   b. a converter   d. a conductor   _____

16. The unit that measures the pressure or force that pushes the flow of electrons forward through a complete electric circuit is called _____.
   a. a watt   c. an ampere
   b. an ohm   d. a volt   _____

17. The unit that measures the number of electrons that flow through a complete electric circuit is called _____.
   a. a watt   c. an ampere
   b. an ohm   d. a volt   _____

18. A measurement of how much electricity is being used in one second is called _____.
   a. a watt   c. an ampere
   b. an ohm   d. a volt   _____

19. A unit that measures the resistance in an electric circuit is called _____.
    a. a watt   c. an ampere
    b. an ohm   d. a volt   _____

20. Normal electric wall sockets that power a paraffin heater are _____ volts.
    a. 9   c. 12
    b. 110   d. 220   _____

21. If you needed to operate a heavy-duty appliance, such as a clothes dryer, you would typically need an outlet with a minimum of _____ volts.
    a. 9   c. 121
    b. 12   d. 220   _____

22. A higher amp rating indicates _____.
    a. a greater number of electrons and a weaker current
    b. a greater number of electrons and a stronger current
    c. fewer electrons and a weaker current
    d. fewer electrons and a stronger current   _____

23. The current for facial and scalp treatments is measured in _____.
    a. watts   c. milliamperes
    b. kilowatts   d. amperes   _____

24. Current will not flow through a conductor unless _____.
    a. the volts are stronger than the ohms
    b. the amps are stronger than the volts
    c. the watts are stronger than the amps
    d. the ohms are stronger than the watts   _____

25. A 75-watt light bulb uses 75 watts of electricity _____.
    a. per minute   c. per hour
    b. per second   d. per day   _____

26. The electricity in your house is measured in _____.
    a. amps per hour   c. kilowatts per hour
    b. milliamperes per hour d. watts per hour   _____

27. What does a light-cured nail enhancement use to harden?
    a. Heat   c. Visible light
    b. Evaporation   d. UV light   _____

28. UV radiation has a shorter wavelength, more _____, and does not penetrate as deeply as visible light.
   a. vibration   c. chemicals
   b. radiation   d. energy   _____

29. Storing heat-curing monomers in a warm place can result in discoloration and _____.
   a. disintegration   c. premature hardening
   b. less penetration   d. longer effectiveness   _____

30. A careless electrical connection and overloaded circuits can result in an electrical shock, a burn, or _____.
   a. power loss   c. excess static
   b. flickering power   d. fire   _____

31. A _____ is a single use safety device designed to provide protection from an electrical overload.
   a. fuse   c. rectifier
   b. circuit breaker   d. converter   _____

32. To reestablish the circuit when a fuse blows, first _____.
   a. check all connections   c. check all insulation
   b. disconnect all appliances d. insert a new fuse   _____

33. A circuit breaker will _____ when the circuit overloads.
   a. reduce power   c. melt
   b. blow out   d. shut off   _____

34. GFCI stands for _____.
   a. General Faradic Current Interrupter
   b. Ground Fault Circuit Interrupter
   c. Ground Fault Circuit Insurer
   d. Greater Frequency Current Interrupter   _____

35. Which of the following certifies the safety of electrical appliances?
   a. Underwriters Laboratories
   b. Better Business Bureau
   c. OSHA
   d. Electrical Engineers Organization   _____

36. Which connection on an electric plug supplies current to the circuit?
   a. The ground connection   c. The live connection
   b. The safety connection   d. The open connection   _____

37. What is the main purpose of the third prong on a three-prong plug?
    a. To provide an additional ground
    b. To serve as a reserve ground
    c. To prevent disconnection
    d. To increase the electrical flow   _____

38. All electrical appliances used should be _____ certified.
    a. UV   c. EA
    b. UL   d. EE   _____

39. It is recommended that you use how many plugs per outlet?
    a. None   c. One
    b. Two   d. Four   _____

40. If an electrical plug does not fit into an outlet, you should _____.
    a. use pliers to snap off the extra ground prong
    b. cut the plug off and insert the exposed wires into the outlet
    c. bend the plug as necessary to make it fit
    d. find a different outlet that accommodates the plug   _____

41. Electricity is a flow of _____.
    a. neutrons   c. electrons
    b. protons   d. positrons   _____

42. Most _____ are good conductors.
    a. woods   c. rocks
    b. metals   d. plastics   _____

43. A typical flashlight runs on _____.
    a. direct current   c. faradic current
    b. alternating current   d. tesla current   _____

44. Car batteries are _____ volts.
    a. 9   c. 110
    b. 12   d. 220   _____

45. Avoid contact with _____ and metal surfaces when using electrical appliances.
    a. plastic   c. rubber
    b. cement   d. water   _____

CHAPTER 13: MANICURING

1. The list of services that you are legally allowed to perform in your specialty as set forth by the regulatory agency in your state is known as your _____.
    a. realm of practice
    c. scope of practice
    b. state practice guidelines
    d. safety practice oversight   _____

2. It is recommended that you use a _____ bulb in the lamp attached to your manicure table.
    a. 20- to 40-watt incandescent
    b. 40- to 60-watt incandescent
    c. 75- to 100-watt incandescent
    d. 12-watt incandescent   _____

3. The Universal Precautions include guidelines in the use of gloves, masks, and eyewear when contact with blood or _____ is a possibility.
    a. seasonal viruses
    c. dirty tools
    b. contaminated objects
    d. body secretions   _____

4. The fingerbowl is used for soaking the client's fingers in warm water to soften the skin and can be made of plastic, _____, or glass.
    a. wood
    c. acrylic
    b. metal
    d. cement   _____

5. Disinfection containers must _____ to ensure disinfectant solution does not become contaminated.
    a. be made of glass
    c. have a lid
    b. be made of plastic
    d. hold two quarts   _____

6. What should you use to cover the client's arm cushion?
    a. Nothing
    c. White paper
    b. A clean towel
    d. Plastic wrap   _____

7. Electric mitts are used to _____.
    a. inhibit the penetration of conditioning ingredients
    b. provide for the ultimate relaxation of the client
    c. keep the client's hands cool and stable
    d. prepare the hands or feet for massage   _____

8. Multiple use and single use tools used to perform nail services are called _____.
    a. supplies
    c. equipment
    b. materials
    d. implements   _____

9. Disposable implements _____.
   a. are generally made of stainless steel
   b. are generally made of nickel-plated metal
   c. must be thrown away after a single use
   d. must be thrown away after several uses _____

10. Tweezers are multitask implements that can be used to _____.
    a. trim the cuticle of the nail
    b. lift small bits of debris from the nail plate
    c. trim the free edge of the nail
    d. place cotton between the toes _____

11. Which of the following is used to shorten the nail plate quickly and effectively?
    a. Nail clippers   c. Nail file
    b. Nippers   d. Metal pusher _____

12. How many complete sets of implements should a professional nail technician have on hand?
    a. One   c. Three
    b. Two   d. Five or more _____

13. The rule of thumb with nail files is _____.
    a. the lower the grit, the smaller the abrasive particles
    b. the lower the grit, the more aggressive its action
    c. the higher the grit, the larger the abrasive particles
    d. the higher the grit, the more aggressive its action _____

14. A buffer with a grit of 180 is considered to be a _____.
    a. medium-grit abrasive   c. coarse abrasive
    b. fine-grit abrasive   d. minimal abrasive _____

15. Fine-grit abrasives are recommended for all but which of the following?
    a. Buffing the nail   c. Shortening the nail
    b. Removing fine scratches d. Polishing the nail _____

16. Soaps acts as an infection-control tool during the preservice hand-washing procedure and is known to remove over _____ percent of pathogenic microbes from the hands, if performed properly.
    a. 30   c. 50
    b. 70   d. 90 _____

17. What are the two basic types of polish removers?
    a. Alcohol and peroxide   c. Lanolin and glycerin
    b. Acetone and non-acetone   d. Soap and acetone   _____

18. Nail creams are designed to _____.
    a. hold subdermal moisture in the skin
    b. absorb into the nail plate
    c. make the nail plate more flexible
    d. strengthen the skin around the nail   _____

19. Which of the following is designed to loosen and dissolve
    dead tissue on the nail plate so it can be more easily and
    thoroughly removed from the nail plate?
    a. Nail oil   c. Nail dehydrator
    b. Nail bleach   d. Cuticle remover   _____

20. Protein hardener is commonly composed of what two
    ingredients?
    a. Clear polish and collagen
    b. Colored polish and collagen
    c. Clear polish and formaldehyde
    d. Colored polish and formaldehyde   _____

21. Nail plate hardeners contain methylene glycol, an ingredient
    that creates _____ between the keratin strands that
    make up the natural nail.
    a. ridges or furrows   c. bridges or cross-links
    b. connections   d. gap closers   _____

22. Compared to methylene glycol hardeners, dimethyl urea
    hardeners _____.
    a. work more slowly
    b. cause more adverse skin reactions
    c. overharden the nails
    d. are less convenient   _____

23. A base coat creates a colorless layer on the natural nail and
    nail enhancement that promotes _____.
    a. a smoother finish   c. a shinier finish
    b. the adhesion of polish   d. the use of less color   _____

24. It is recommended that you work to get your basic manicure
    procedure to _____ before you leave your school
    environment.
    a. 25–30 minutes   c. 45–60 minutes
    b. 30–45 minutes   d. 60–90 minutes   _____

25. The _____ nail is completely straight across the free edge, with no rounding at the outside edges.
   a. round
   b. oval
   c. square
   d. squoval

   _____

26. A _____ nail is one with a square free edge that is rounded off at the corner edges.
   a. round
   b. pointed
   c. square
   d. squoval

   _____

27. Lighter shades are generally recommended for which seasons?
   a. Spring and summer
   b. Summer and autumn
   c. Autumn and winter
   d. Winter and spring

   _____

28. What is the recommended method for mixing nail polish in the bottle?
   a. Stirring it with the nail polish brush
   b. Shaking the bottle from side to side
   c. Rolling the bottle between your palms
   d. Shaking the bottle up and down

   _____

29. The most successful nail polish application is achieved by applying how many coats?
   a. One
   b. Two
   c. Three
   d. Four

   _____

30. A man's manicure is performed using the same procedures as described in the basic manicure, though you omit the colored polish and _____.
   a. apply dehydrator for a dull finish
   b. exfoliate the eponychium
   c. buff with a high-shine buffer
   d. apply a spa hand mask

   _____

31. The manipulation of the soft tissues of the body is called
   _____.
   a. chiropractic
   b. aromatherapy
   c. a manicure
   d. massage

   _____

32. Which type of massage is also known as kneading?
   a. Tapotement
   b. Friction
   c. Petrissage
   d. Effleurage

   _____

33. Results-oriented spa manicures are sometimes called
   _____.
   a. pedicures
   b. treatment manicures
   c. mani-pedicures
   d. medi-manicures

   _____

34. Which of the following involves the use of highly concentrated, nonoily, and volatile essential oils?
   a. Aromatherapy
   b. Pedicure
   c. Effleurage
   d. Petrissage ____

35. Paraffin wax treatments are designed to trap moisture in the skin while the _____ encourages skin pores to accept its benefits.
   a. lotion
   b. chemicals
   c. wax
   d. heat ____

36. Avoid paraffin treatments on anyone who has _____ or skin irritations such as cuts, burns, rashes, warts, or eczema.
   a. edema
   b. high stress
   c. diabetes
   d. impaired circulation ____

37. _____ is a petroleum by-product that has excellent sealing properties (barrier qualities) to hold moisture in the skin.
   a. Lanolin
   b. Glycerin
   c. Paraffin
   d. Mineral oil ____

38. When performing a basic manicure, it is recommended that you start with the _____.
   a. little finger on the client's left hand
   b. little finger on the client's right hand
   c. thumb on the client's left hand
   d. thumb on the client's right hand ____

39. The second step in a preservice procedure is to _____.
   a. clean implements and place in disinfectant solution
   b. put on gloves to prevent contamination of implements
   c. rinse implements and wash with soap, a nail brush, and warm water
   d. rinse away all traces of soap with warm running water ____

40. In preparation for a hand massage, apply massage lotion or cream and distribute enough to allow movement across the skin without resistance or _____.
   a. opposition
   b. chafing
   c. skin wrinkling
   d. skin drag ____

41. The third step in a postservice procedure is to _____.
   a. escort client to front desk and schedule next appointment
   b. advise clients regarding home maintenance
   c. condition the client's hands
   d. thank the client and give him/her an appointment card ____

42. The drying time after a nail polish application should be _____ minimum.
    a. 5 minutes
    b. 10 minutes
    c. 15 minutes
    d. 20 minutes
    _____

43. How long should you allow the paraffin to remain on the client's hands during a paraffin wax treatment?
    a. 3–5 seconds
    b. 3–5 minutes
    c. 5–10 minutes
    d. 10–20 minutes
    _____

CHAPTER 14: PEDICURING

1. Cosmetic services performed on the feet by a licensed nail technician or cosmetologist that include trimming, shaping, exfoliating, polishing toenails, and massage are called _____.
   a. manicures
   b. pedicures
   c. aromatherapy
   d. reflexology ___

2. Pedicures create client loyalty, produce considerable income, and can be important _____ for many clients.
   a. medical treatment
   b. self-esteem building treatment
   c. emotional therapy
   d. preventive health services ___

3. Shaving the legs within 24 hours of having a pedicure increases the risk of _____, which causes tiny unseen openings in the skin that may allow entry by pathogenic microbes.
   a. macrotrauma
   b. irritation
   c. microtrauma
   d. infection ___

4. Which term refers to all of the permanent tools used to perform nail services that are not implements?
   a. Equipment
   b. Materials
   c. Supplies
   d. Pedicure products ___

5. When preparing the pedicure foot bath, it is recommended that you fill it with _____ water.
   a. cold
   b. cool
   c. hot
   d. warm ___

6. Some fully plumbed whirlpool baths are _____ and connected to a drain.
   a. portable and flexible
   b. permanently plumbed to hot and cold water
   c. filled using a hose to run water into the bath
   d. manually filled ___

7. Electric foot mitts are designed to _____.
   a. add a special touch to a pedicure
   b. slow the penetration of the conditioning ingredients
   c. help keep the client's feet from feeling cool
   d. create a stimulating effect ___

8. Toenail clippers have a _____ space between the jaws, allowing them to cut thicker nails.
   a. curved
   b. jagged
   c. wider
   d. narrower ___

9. Which implement has a small, scoop-shaped end?
   a. Nail rasp   c. Nipper
   b. Toenail clipper   d. Curette   _____

10. Only curettes with _____ are safe and appropriate for nail technicians to use.
    a. replaceable blades   c. dull edges
    b. permanent blades   d. sharp edges   _____

11. For most clients, a _____ nail file is recommended for pedicures.
    a. medium-grit   c. fine-grit
    b. grit abrasive   d. grit-free   _____

12. Foot files or paddles are designed to reduce and smooth _____.
    a. warts   c. skin irritations
    b. lesions   d. thicker foot calluses _____

13. Which implement is used to trim tags of dead skin?
    a. Toenail clipper   c. Nail rasp
    b. Nipper   d. Foot paddle   _____

14. You should not use metal pushers or sharp implements on clients who have _____.
    a. skin irritation   c. any chronic disease
    b. had a recent illness d. edema   _____

15. A spa pedicure usually lasts for about _____ minutes.
    a. 20–30   c. 45–60
    b. 30–45   d. 60–90   _____

16. Toe separators are used when _____.
    a. massaging the feet   c. exfoliating the feet
    b. polishing the toenails d. clipping the toenails _____

17. The disposable slippers provided for clients who have not worn open-toe shoes and want to avoid smudging their newly applied toenail polish are typically made of _____.
    a. rubber or cotton   c. paper or foam
    b. paper or plastic   d. rubber or plastic _____

18. Which type of product is put into the water in a pedicure bath to soften the skin on the feet?
    a. Foot soaks   c. Scrubs
    b. Essential oils   d. Masks   _____

19. Exfoliating scrubs are usually _____ that contain an abrasive as the exfoliating agent.
    a. oil-based creams
    b. water-based lotions
    c. crystallized creams
    d. oil-based breams
    _____

20. Masks are commonly made with mineral clays, moisturizing agents, skin softeners, aromatherapy oils, and _____.
    a. skin sloughers
    b. skin scrubs
    c. beneficial extracts
    d. skin antiseptics
    _____

21. Callus softener products are applied _____.
    a. directly to the callus
    b. by mixing with water in a pedicure bath
    c. spraying on entire foot with a mister
    d. by mixing with a softening lotion
    _____

22. Which abbreviation refers to a licensed nail technician or cosmetologist who has taken advanced education to learn to perform safe pedicures on podiatry patients?
    a. NMC
    b. INTA
    c. MNT
    d. EPA
    _____

23. Treatments that require multiple appointments are referred to as _____.
    a. a grouping
    b. a series
    c. successive services
    d. a collection
    _____

24. Appointments to ensure lower calluses should be scheduled _____.
    a. weekly
    b. daily
    c. monthly
    d. biweekly
    _____

25. A typical callus reduction appointment includes a soak application, a reduction product application and treatment, _____, and dismissal.
    a. nail polish application
    b. foot massage
    c. a lotion application
    d. an antiseptic application
    _____

26. A client going through a callus reduction process will typically require about _____ visits.
    a. 2–3
    b. 4–6
    c. 8–10
    d. 12–15
    _____

27. The typical method for applying paraffin from the bath is to dip and re-dip the hands or feet _____ times into the larger paraffin bath.
    a. 1–2
    b. 2–3
    c. 3–4
    d. 4–6
    _____

28. The massage performed during a pedicure service is predominantly _____.
    a. effleurage
    b. petrissage
    c. tapotement
    d. vibration

    _____

29. Reflexology is a unique method of applying pressure with the thumb and index fingers to the hands and feet and demonstrates _____.
    a. healing of chronic illness
    b. healing of back pain
    c. control of foot pain
    d. health benefits

    _____

30. Hot stones are used in pedicures to provide a deep, penetrating, and comforting heat that enhances relaxation and _____.
    a. ability to sleep
    b. circulation
    c. stimulation
    d. blood flow reduction

    _____

31. Salons must always use an EPA-registered hospital disinfectant that is labeled a broad spectrum _____, viricide, and fungicide.
    a. bactericide
    b. tuberculocide
    c. germicide
    d. antibiotic

    _____

32. Ergonomics in pedicuring focuses on _____.
    a. the technician's body positioning
    b. the products used
    c. water temperature
    d. massage techniques

    _____

33. Generally when performing a foot massage the foot should be gently grasped _____.
    a. just above the ankle
    b. by the heal
    c. between the thumb and the fingers
    d. just below the toes

    _____

34. When performing a pedicure, a _____ is used to gently remove and loose and dead tissue.
    a. nail brush
    b. wooden pusher
    c. nail clipper
    d. curette

    _____

35. Curettes must always be used with the bowl of the curette _____ the skin.
    a. horizontal to
    b. toward the skin
    c. away from the skin
    d. directly opposite from

    _____

36. Nail technicians can _____.
    a. prevent ingrown nails
    b. can treat ingrown nails
    c. cut and trim calluses
    d. cannot cut or trim calluses

    _____

37. _____ is a traditional release in massage.
    a. Feathering   c. Reflexology
    b. Patting lightly   d. Gently squeezing   ____

38. After a pedicure, what is the first step prior to applying the base coat?
    a. Using polish remover to remove oils and lotion from the nails.
    b. Asking client to put on pedicure slippers.
    c. Applying toe separators.
    d. Applying moisturizer.   ____

39. What is the purpose of a callus?
    a. A callus has no purpose
    b. To prevent foot dehydration
    c. To protect the underlying skin from irritation
    d. To help regulate the foot temperature   ____

40. When using a curette to remove loose debris from the nail plate, it is recommended that you use a _____ motion.
    a. up-and-down   c. side-to-side
    b. scooping   d. circular   ____

41. The _____ toenail is usually the most challenging to trim.
    a. big   c. little
    b. middle   d. second   ____

42. Massaging the leg is not recommended for clients with severe hypertension or circulatory problems because it _____.
    a. promotes inflammation   c. increases circulation
    b. inhibits inflammation   d. decreases circulation   ____

43. The basic pedicure includes a foot massage and not a leg massage due to time constraints and the fact that it is considered to be _____.
    a. inappropriate   c. a special service addition
    b. excessive   d. inefficient and costly   ____

44. Foot care mask ingredients are used to cleanse, exfoliate, tighten, tone, hydrate, and _____ the skin.
    a. roughen   c. loosen
    b. nourish   d. circulate   ____

45. When performing a pedicure, it is recommended that you _____ as you work.
    a. lean forward toward client
    b. keep your body relaxed and unstrained
    c. stretch to reach your client's feet
    d. keep your back rigid and firm   ____

CHAPTER 15: ELECTRIC FILING

1. The motor of a micromotor machine is located _____.
   a. inside the handpiece
   b. inside the base box
   c. in a separate area outside the machine
   d. inside the head   ____

2. Battery-operated micromotors are small, compact, and powerful, _____.
   a. but more difficult to use
   b. and are easier to use
   c. but some have much less torque
   d. and have even more torque   ____

3. What is a significant clue in determining the authenticity of a micromotor machine?
   a. Its price   c. Its appearance
   b. Its packaging   d. Its power   ____

4. Electric files purchased at craft, hobby, and tool stores are not recommended for use in the salon because they are manufactured for use on glass, wood, and ceramics and can damage the natural and artificial nail because of _____.
   a. the grit   c. the lack of power
   b. the amount of vibration   d. the lack of torque   ____

5. The speed of electric files is measured in _____.
   a. RPM   c. RPH
   b. MPH   d. MPM   ____

6. Which term refers to the tightness of the inside of the shank where the bit fits into the handpiece?
   a. Mandrel   c. Tolerance
   b. Chuck   d. Torque   ____

7. When selecting an electric file, the handpiece should weigh approximately 4 to 6 ounces, should be comfortable in your hand, and _____.
   a. have strong vibration   c. have minimal grip
   b. have virtually no vibration   d. have a rigid grip   ____

8. The power in the machine or its ability to keep turning when applying pressure during filing is known as _____.
   a. tolerance   c. velocity
   b. rapidity   d. torque   ____

9. Most manufacturers can service and return your electric file within _____.
   a. 2–3 days
   b. 12–14 days
   c. 15–20 days
   d. 7–10 days
   _____

10. Most manufacturers will fix or replace a malfunctioning electric file within _____ of purchase at no cost to you.
   a. 6 months
   b. 1 year
   c. 3 years
   d. 5 years
   _____

11. Concentric bits are commonly referred to as being _____.
   a. top-heavy
   b. bottom-heavy
   c. centered
   d. unsteady
   _____

12. Wobbling bits can harm the electric file or cause damage to the client's nails and may cause the nail professional to develop _____.
   a. a CTD
   b. a MNT
   c. a STD
   d. an UNC
   _____

13. Which term refers to the number of abrasive particles per square inch on an electric file?
   a. Edge
   b. Finishing
   c. Grit
   d. Shank
   _____

14. The long, slender cuts or grooves found on a carbide bit are known as _____.
   a. mandrels
   b. flutes
   c. shanks
   d. chucks
   _____

15. Grooves carved into the nail by filing with bits at the incorrect angle are known as _____.
   a. flutes
   b. shanks
   c. mandrels
   d. rings of fire
   _____

16. Traditional carbides must be used from the right to left with the machine in _____.
   a. forward rotation
   b. backward rotation
   c. clockwise rotation
   d. counterclockwise rotation
   _____

17. An UNC bit is recommended for tight spaces such as under the nail, sidewalls, and for making _____ in nails.
   a. grooves
   b. wavy ridges
   c. designer holes
   d. corrugations
   _____

18. Cone-shaped bits are slim, long, tapered, and _____ so they can be used at the cuticle and underneath the nail.
   a. rounded
   b. long
   c. smoothed
   d. pointed
   _____

19. Backfill bits come in two sizes: small _____ the size of a barrel bit and medium _____ the size of a barrel bit.
    a. 1/4; 1/2   c. 1/8; 1/4
    b. 1/3; 1/2   d. 1/2; 3/4   _____

20. High-shine bits are commonly made of _____, cotton, or soft leather material.
    a. natural chamois   c. neutral nylon
    b. heavy linen   d. fiberglass   _____

21. High-shine bits are sometimes called _____.
    a. buffer bits   c. synthetic bits
    b. needle bits   d. pedicure bits   _____

22. Pedicure bits are used on _____ speed.
    a. slow   c. medium to high
    b. slow to medium   d. high   _____

23. Sanding bands are made of _____.
    a. paper   c. linen
    b. chamois   d. silk   _____

24. Sanding bands are generally used for shortening and shaping the top surface of the nails, _____, and filing calluses on the feet.
    a. adding moisture to the nail plate
    b. removing a gel sealant
    c. filing away unwanted lesions
    d. removing natural oils   _____

25. The bullet bit is a small, slender bit that is available in a flat-topped or round-tipped version and is similar to the _____ bit.
    a. needle   c. UNC
    b. football-shaped   d. French fill   _____

26. A long, slender carbide bit that has been made for drilling a hole into the free edge of a nail enhancement to attach nail jewelry is known as _____.
    a. a diamond bit   c. an arbor band
    b. a needle bit   d. a jewelry bit   _____

27. Replace a dirty metal bit with a _____ as part of routine cleanup in between clients.
    a. blank   c. clean bit
    b. cotton strip   d. tissue   _____

28. When practicing with your electric file, it is recommended that you glue a nail tip on a dowel or round clothespin and hold the dowel as you would hold a _____.
    a. hammer   c. piece of fruit
    b. client's finger   d. paintbrush   ____

29. It is recommended that you use the _____ as the fulcrum finger when balancing your hands while using an electric file.
    a. thumb   c. middle finger
    b. index finger   d. pinky finger   ____

30. When performing cuticle work, it is recommended that you set your electric file to _____ speed.
    a. medium   c. slow
    b. fast   d. turbo   ____

31. There are four types of carbide bits including one-way, cross-cut, pointed flutes that cut in both directions, and _____.
    a. conventional   c. regular
    b. traditional   d. exotic   ____

32. A shorter, cone-shaped bit that is designed with a flat top and can be used to shape the top surface of the nail and to cut maintenance on small nails at a flat angle is known as _____.
    a. a tapered barrel bit   c. small barreled bit
    b. a large barrel bit   d. cuticle safety bit   ____

33. When performing finishing work with the electric file, it is recommended that you move from _____ bits.
    a. coarser to finer   c. coarser to finer to coarser
    b. finer to coarser   d. finer to coarser to finer   ____

34. When using an electric file, buffing oils should be used _____.
    a. generously   c. never
    b. sparingly   d. as requested   ____

35. Electric filing on foot calluses needs to be done when the foot is _____.
    a. unwashed   c. damp
    b. wet   d. dry   ____

36. When practicing cuticle work, place the bit at the cuticle area, holding the bit a slight angle so that the top and at least _____ percent of the bit is making contact with the nail.
    a. 50   c. 60
    b. 70   d. 80   ____

37. When electric filing, the smallest dust particles are caused by
_____.
   a. carbide bits
   b. diamond bits
   c. sanders or sleeves
   d. rings of fire   _____

38. To reduce the amount of heat created when using an electric
file, it is recommended that you _____.
   a. adjust the speed of the machine slightly higher
   b. use consistent pressure with the bit
   c. press down harder
   d. leave the bit in the same place on the nail   _____

39. The term _____ refers to the bit catching the skin
around the nail during filing.
   a. "rings of fire"
   b. "grabbing"
   c. "stabbing"
   d. "clocking"   _____

40. The bit on an electric file _____.
   a. moves side-to-side
   b. moves up and down
   c. turns counterclockwise
   d. turns clockwise   _____

41. To prevent grabbing, it is recommended that you keep the
bit parallel to the nail, angle the finger to file the sides of the
nail, and use bits with _____ such as safety style bits.
   a. level
   b. straight
   c. rounded
   d. pointed   _____

42. Common causes of free-edge separation include product
breakdown, the client's treatment of the nails, and _____.
   a. product use
   b. improper filing
   c. product age
   d. exposure to the elements   _____

43. When a nail enhancement ages with wear and becomes
brittle and develops tiny cracks, it is called _____.
   a. rings of fire
   b. microshattering
   c. product breakdown
   d. microtrauma   _____

44. When using an electric file, it is important to keep the
bit _____.
   a. straight up and down
   b. parallel to the nail
   c. at an angle to the nail
   d. diagonally across the free edge   _____

45. When washing metal file bits prior to disinfection, it is
recommended that you rinse them with _____.
   a. warm water
   b. hot water
   c. cold water
   d. acetone   _____

CHAPTER 16: NAIL TIPS AND WRAPS

1. Plastic, premolded nails shaped from a tough polymer made from acrylonitrile butadiene styrene (ABS) plastic are commonly known as _____.
   a. nail wraps
   b. nail tips
   c. fabric wraps
   d. paper wraps
   _____

2. A layer of any kind of nail enhancement product that is applied over the tip for added strength is known as _____.
   a. an overlay
   b. a repair patch
   c. a stress strip
   d. a strengthener
   _____

3. In addition to the basic materials found on a manicuring table, nail tips, abrasive boards, a buffer block, nail tip adhesive, nail dehydrator, and _____ are needed for a nail tip application.
   a. toenail clippers
   b. resin activator
   c. a tip cutter
   d. linen strips
   _____

4. _____ is used to remove surface moisture and tiny amounts of oil left on the natural plate.
   a. Nail dehydrator
   b. Nail wrap resin
   c. Nail cream
   d. Acetone
   _____

5. The point where the free edge of the natural nail meets the tip and where the tip is adhered to the nail is known as the _____.
   a. shallow depression
   b. stress point
   c. position stop
   d. adhesion point
   _____

6. When fitting tips to your client, make sure that the tips chosen cover the nail plate from _____.
   a. cuticle to free edge
   b. sidewall to sidewall
   c. lunula to free edge
   d. cuticle to fingertip
   _____

7. If you do not have a tip that fits the client's nail exactly, it is recommended that you use a slightly _____ tip and bevel it to fit.
   a. longer
   b. shorter
   c. narrower
   d. larger
   _____

8. The bonding agent used to secure the nail tip to the natural nail is called _____.
   a. nail tip dehydrator
   b. liquid adhering drops
   c. nail tip adhesive
   d. gel bonding agent
   _____

9. Once nail tips are applied, the contact area will need to be
_____ with an abrasive, so that the tip blends smoothly
with the natural nail.
a. reduced
b. expanded
c. strengthened
d. softened
_____

10. Any method of securing a layer of fabric or paper on and
around the nail tip to ensure its strength and durability is
called _____.
a. an overlap
b. adhesion application
c. a nail tip
d. a nail wrap
_____

11. Wrap resins are made from _____ and are closely
related to those used to create other types of nail
enhancements.
a. monomer
b. cyanoacrylate
c. polymer
d. methocrylate
_____

12. _____ wraps are made from a closely woven, heavy
material.
a. Silk
b. Linen
c. Nylon
d. Fiberglass
_____

13. A fabric wrap is the most popular type of nail wrap because of
its _____.
a. application
b. durability
c. flexibility
d. cost
_____

14. _____ wraps are made from a very thin synthetic mesh
with a loose weave.
a. Silk
b. Linen
c. Nylon
d. Fiberglass
_____

15. _____ wraps are made from a thin natural material with
a tight weave that becomes transparent with wrap resin is
applied.
a. Silk
b. Linen
c. Nylon
d. Fiberglass
_____

16. Paper wraps are _____ and very simple to use.
a. durable
b. strong
c. temporary
d. heavy
_____

17. Another term for a wrap resin accelerator is _____.
a. strengthener
b. catalyst
c. adhesive
d. activator
_____

18. A wrap resin accelerator acts as the dryer that _____ the hardening process of the wrap resin or adhesive overlay.
    a. moderates
    b. speeds up
    c. slows up
    d. controls
    _____

19. Activators are available in several different forms including brush-on bottle, pump spray-on, and _____.
    a. mister
    b. drops
    c. powder
    d. aerosol
    _____

20. In addition to the basic materials on the manicuring table, you will need adhesive-backed fabric, small scissors, wrap resin, wrap resin accelerator, a nail buffer, and _____ to perform a nail wrap application.
    a. a small piece of plastic
    b. nail extension forms
    c. fingernail clippers
    d. nail nippers
    _____

21. Structurally correcting the nail wrap enhancement to ensure its strength, shape, and durability is commonly referred to as _____.
    a. a fill
    b. a rebalance
    c. a backfill
    d. a repair
    _____

22. No Light Gels have the same chemical composition as wrap systems with wrap resin and can be used with a _____ activator to harden or cure the adhesive.
    a. spray-on
    b. drop-on
    c. brush-on
    d. powdered
    _____

23. When cutting a stress strip, it should measure _____ in length.
    a. $\frac{1}{4}$"
    b. $\frac{1}{16}$"
    c. $\frac{1}{32}$"
    d. $\frac{1}{8}$"
    _____

24. A _____ is a piece of fabric cut to completely cover a crack or break in the nail.
    a. stress strip
    b. repair patch
    c. backfill patch
    d. maintenance strip
    _____

25. Fabric wraps are removed by first immersing the entire enhancement into a small bowl filled with _____.
    a. polish remover
    b. resin softener
    c. acetone
    d. cyanoacrylate
    _____

26. After the Preservice Procedure, the first step in a Nail Wrap Application Procedure is to _____.
    a. remove existing polish
    b. lightly buff the nail plate
    c. push back the eponychium
    d. apply a nail dehydrator ___

27. In a *fabric wrap maintenance procedure,* the buffing dust is removed with _____.
    a. a damp, cotton cloth
    b. an aerosol spray
    c. a dry, lint-free cloth
    d. a dry, nylon nail brush ___

28. Nail tips should be worn with _____.
    a. an overlay
    b. nail hardener
    c. nail polish
    d. an adhesive layer ___

29. In the *nail tip removal procedure,* the natural nail is gently buffed with a fine buffer to remove any _____.
    a. remaining nail polish
    b. natural oils
    c. nail tip particles
    d. adhesive residue ___

30. After removing the cuticle during a *nail tip application procedure,* buff over the nail plate with a medium/fine abrasive to _____.
    a. rough the nail plate
    b. remove the shine
    c. thicken the nail plate
    d. improve the shine ___

31. In a *nail tip application procedure,* apply _____ to remove surface moisture and tiny amounts of oil left on the natural nail plate.
    a. nail enamel
    b. polish remover
    c. nail dehydrator
    d. adhesive remover ___

32. When applying the adhesive during a *nail tip application procedure,* place the adhesive _____.
    a. along the free edge
    c. to the entire nail plate
    b. where the tip will be placed
    d. to the lunula ___

33. In a *nail wrap application procedure,* when is the wrap material cut to the approximate width and shape of the nail plate?
    a. After applying wrap resin
    b. Before selecting the nail tip
    c. After applying wrap resin activator
    d. Before removing the wrap backing ___

34. In a *nail wrap application procedure,* the resin is applied to all 10 fingers beginning on the left hand with the _____.
    a. index finger
    b. pinky finger
    c. thumb
    d. middle finger ___

35. In a *nail wrap application procedure,* once the fabric is secure
on the nail, use small scissors to trim the fabric _____
inch away from the sidewalls and the free edge.
   a. 1/8
   b. 1/4
   c. 1/16
   d. 1/32 ____

36. In a *nail wrap application procedure,* to seal the free edge
and prevent lifting and tip separation, _____.
   a. apply a second coat of wrap resin
   b. apply a nail hardener product
   c. apply a second layer of wrap material
   d. buff seam to a fine finish ____

37. In a *nail tip application procedure,* after shaping and refining
the nail wrap, _____ is applied before buffing.
   a. nail cream
   b. cuticle cream
   c. nail oil
   d. nail polish ____

38. Which common household item may be used to press the
fabric wrap onto the nail plate during a *nail wrap application
procedure?*
   a. A pencil eraser
   b. A plastic sandwich bag
   c. A plastic spoon
   d. A Popsicle stick ____

39. It is recommended that you use _____ to remove a
client's nail polish during a *fabric wrap maintenance
procedure.*
   a. acetone polish remover
   b. warm soap and water
   c. nonacetone polish remover
   d. warm cuticle oil ____

40. When removing fabric wraps, the acetone level in the small
glass bowl should be approximately _____ the nail
wraps.
   a. ½" above
   b. ¼" below
   c. level with
   d. ¼" above ____

41. Linen wraps are _____ and require a colored polish to
cover it completely.
   a. translucent
   b. reflective
   c. transparent
   d. opaque ____

42. A _____ wrap is lightweight and has a smooth
appearance when applied to the nail.
   a. linen
   b. fiberglass
   c. silk
   d. paper ____

43. When applying nail tips, an abrasive should be used to shape the free edges of the natural nails to match the shape of the nail tip to the _____.
    a. half moon
    b. stop point
    c. free edge
    d. full well
    _____

44. Cutting a nail tip with any tool other than a professional tip cutter will weaken it and cause it to _____.
    a. crack
    b. lift
    c. loosen
    d. soften
    _____

45. _____ is the term used when a nail enhancement needs to be serviced after 2 or more weeks from the initial application.
    a. Repair
    b. Upkeep
    c. Support
    d. Maintenance
    _____

CHAPTER 17: MONOMER LIQUID AND POLYMER POWDER NAIL ENHANCEMENTS

1. All nail enhancement products are based almost entirely on ingredients that come from the _____ family.
   - a. synthetic fiber
   - b. acrylic
   - c. synthetic textile
   - d. plastic
   ____

2. The "poly" in polymer means _____.
   - a. one
   - b. units
   - c. many
   - d. few
   ____

3. Which of the following is not one of the three versions of monomer liquid used in the nail industry?
   - a. Odorless monomer liquid
   - b. Ethyl methacrylate
   - c. Ethyl acrylic
   - d. Methyl methacrylate
   ____

4. Polymer powder is made using a special chemical reaction called _____.
   - a. plasticization
   - b. crystallization
   - c. excoriation
   - d. polymerization
   ____

5. Ethyl methacrylate monomer liquid is commonly referred to as _____.
   - a. EMA
   - b. EML
   - c. EMM
   - d. EMML
   ____

6. Methyl methacrylate (MMA) is not recommended for use on nails and is _____ in some states.
   - a. not sold
   - b. not available
   - c. extremely expensive
   - d. not legal
   ____

7. MMA nail products do not adhere well to the nail plate requiring the nail technician to _____ the surface of the nail.
   - a. shred or etch
   - b. smooth or shine
   - c. file or buff
   - d. polish or shine
   ____

8. MMA creates the hardest and _____ nail enhancements.
   - a. most flexible
   - b. most rigid
   - c. smoothest
   - d. most desirable
   ____

9. MMA _____ in product removers.
   - a. softens easily
   - b. dissolves quickly
   - c. does not dissolve well
   - d. requires additional chemicals
   ____

10. MMA is a widely used monomer with a long history of safe use in medical and _____ products.
    a. dental   c. prosthesis
    b. implant   d. hearing aid   _____

11. When monomer liquid is picked up by a brush and mixed with polymer powder, it creates what is known as a _____.
    a. gleam   c. mound
    b. curette   d. bead   _____

12. A catalyst is an additive designed to _____ chemical reactions.
    a. slow down   c. speed up
    b. neutralize   d. stabilize   _____

13. The initiators found in polymer powder, when activated by a catalyst will spring into action and cause monomer molecules to permanently link together into _____.
    a. short polymer chains   c. a single monomer
    b. long polymer chains   d. polymerized molecules   _____

14. Compared to acne treatments, nail powders contain _____.
    a. the same percentage of benzoyl peroxide
    b. more benzoyl peroxide
    c. less benzoyl peroxide
    d. no benzoyl peroxide   _____

15. It is recommended that you mix $1\frac{1}{2}$ parts monomer liquid with 1 part polymer powder to create a _____ bead.
    a. medium   c. dry
    b. wet   d. damp   _____

16. The amount of monomer liquid and polymer powder used to create a bead is called the _____.
    a. mid-ratio   c. bead equation
    b. mix speed   d. mix ratio   _____

17. In general, _____ beads are the ideal mix ratio for working with monomer liquids and polymer powders.
    a. wet   c. medium
    b. dry   d. heavy   _____

18. Nail _____ remove surface moisture and tiny amounts of oil left on the natural nail plate.
    a. moisturizers   c. creams
    b. dehydrators   d. dryers   _____

19. Nail dehydrator should be applied liberally to the _____ only.
    a. nail plate
    b. nail bed
    c. eponychium
    d. free edge
    _____

20. Nail _____ is used on the natural nail prior to product application to assist in adhesion.
    a. dehydrator
    b. base
    c. polish
    d. primer
    _____

21. When applying an acid-based nail primer, it is recommended that you use _____.
    a. a light dotting action
    b. long, narrow strokes
    c. slow, wide strokes
    d. a circular stroke
    _____

22. A medium-grit abrasive is not recommended for _____.
    a. initial shaping of the nail
    b. refining the overall surface shape of the nail
    c. smoothing the surface before buffing
    d. finish filing of the nail
    _____

23. Nail forms generally are not made of _____.
    a. mylar
    b. fiberglass
    c. paper
    d. aluminum
    _____

24. Which type of nail form can be disinfected?
    a. Plastic
    b. Paper
    c. Silk
    d. Fiberglass
    _____

25. The special container used to hold the monomer liquid and polymer powder as you work is called a _____.
    a. finger bowl
    b. disposable dish
    c. liquid vial
    d. dappen dish
    _____

26. The best nail brush to use with monomer liquid and polymer powder enhancement products is composed of natural kolinsky, _____, or a blend of both.
    a. sable
    b. mink
    c. bristle
    d. angora
    _____

27. Unused monomer that has been removed from the original container should be _____.
    a. poured back into the original container for use with another client
    b. poured down the drain with the hot water running
    c. poured into an absorbent paper towel and placed in a plastic bag
    d. poured down the drain with the cold water running
    _____

28. When a nail tech files a damaged section of a monomer liquid and polymer powder enhancement and refills it with the appropriate products, it is called a _____.
   a. backfill
   b. rebalance
   c. maintenance service
   d. crack repair _____

29. A dry mix ratio creates a bead that looks _____ on the brush.
   a. frosted
   b. runny
   c. glossy
   d. dark _____

30. Odorless products harden more slowly and create a tacky layer called the _____.
   a. dehydrator layer
   b. obstruction layer
   c. inhibition layer
   d. assistance layer _____

31. The apex of the nail is also known as the _____.
   a. stress area
   b. sidewall
   c. arch
   d. lunula _____

32. The apex is usually what shape?
   a. Oval
   b. Half-moon
   c. Round
   d. Rectangular _____

33. The area where the natural nail grows beyond the finger and becomes the free edge is known as the _____.
   a. sidewall
   b. arch
   c. apex
   d. stress area _____

34. The length of the nail extensions and enhancements should be the same on _____.
   a. all five fingers
   b. the index, middle, and ring fingers
   c. the index and ring fingers
   d. the thumb, middle finger, and pinky _____

35. The C-curve of the nail enhancement depends on the C-curve of the natural nail, which is on average _____ percent.
   a. 20
   b. 25
   c. 30
   d. 35 _____

36. Some manufacturers make a _____ that brushes on to cure the tacky inhibition layer that must be applied immediately after creating the odorless product enhancement.
   a. resin
   b. hydrator
   c. adhesive
   d. dissolver _____

37. Nail artistry with colored polymer powder is limited only
    by _____.
    a. your resources   c. your pocketbook
    b. your imagination   d. the client's wishes   _____

38. When performing a one-color monomer and polymer nail
    enhancement application, it is recommended that you apply
    _____ after using a pusher to push back the
    eponychium and filing to remove the shine.
    a. nail primer   c. nail dehydrator
    b. nail oil   d. cuticle remover   _____

39. When acid-free primer dries on the nail, it will be
    _____.
    a. sticky and dull   c. smooth and dull
    b. sticky and shiny   d. smooth and shiny   _____

40. When performing a one-color monomer and polymer
    enhancement application, it is recommended that the first
    bead of monomer and polymer applied to the nail be
    _____.
    a. dry   c. medium-to-dry
    b. wet   d. medium-to-wet   _____

41. After applying the first bead of product during a monomer
    and polymer enhancement application, you should use the
    _____ of your brush to press and smooth the product.
    a. middle portion   c. tip
    b. base   d. handle   _____

42. To perform a two-color monomer liquid and polymer powder
    nail enhancement with forms, you will need nail dehydrator,
    nail forms, enhancement product, primer, abrasives, brushes,
    and _____.
    a. cuticle nippers   c. overlay product
    b. dappen dishes   d. nail polish   _____

43. Acid based nail primer will dry to a _____.
    a. chalky white   c. dull frost
    b. clear finish   d. dark finish   _____

44. When performing a two-color monomer and polymer
    enhancement application, the application must be _____
    at the cuticle line,
    a. rough   c. thick
    b. flat   d. thin   _____

45. After the application of the two-color monomer and polymer enhancement, it is recommended that you file the underside of the nail extensions and then glide the abrasive over the nail with _____.
    a. long, sweeping strokes   c. a dotting movement
    b. short, brisk strokes   d. small, circular strokes   _____

46. When performing a one-color monomer and polymer enhancement maintenance service, what should you do if there is excessive, loose nail-enhancement product and lifting?
    a. Use a nipper to clip it away.
    b. Use scissors to clip it away.
    c. Soak off the enhancement and start fresh with a new application.
    d. Apply a strengthening layer of product over the existing enhancement.   _____

47. When performing a two-color monomer and polymer nail enhancement, use the tip of the brush to push _____ into place and wipe the edge until a crisp rounded line is achieved.
    a. the product   c. the frown line
    b. the smile line   d. the lunula   _____

48. Which of the following do you need to perform a crack repair on a monomer and polymer enhancement, but not to perform a standard monomer and polymer maintenance service?
    a. Nail forms   c. Nail primer
    b. Monomer liquid   d. Application brushes   _____

49. When performing a monomer and polymer crack repair, you must apply _____ after applying nail dehydrator.
    a. a dry bead of product
    b. a medium bead of product
    c. nail primer to the entire natural nail and existing enhancement
    d. nail primer to any exposed natural nail in the crack   _____

50. When removing monomer and polymer enhancements, the client's nails should soak in the acetone for _____ or as long as needed to remove the enhancement product.
    a. 5–10 minutes   c. 10–20 minutes
    b. 20–30 minutes   d. 30–45 minutes   _____

CHAPTER 18: UV AND LED GELS

1. UV nail enhancement ingredients are part of a subcategory of a chemical family called acrylates and _____.
   a. methacrylates
   b. cyanoacrylates
   c. acrylics
   d. wrap resins
   _____

2. "Oligo" means _____.
   a. many
   b. only one
   c. a few
   d. units
   _____

3. Oligomers are typically thick, gel-like, and _____.
   a. creamy
   b. dry
   c. moist
   d. sticky
   _____

4. The term _____ refers to the type of starting material that is used to create the most common UV gel resins.
   a. "acrylic"
   b. "methacrylate"
   c. "urethane"
   d. "resin"
   _____

5. UV gel resins react when exposed to the gel's recommended UV light because of a chemical called a _____.
   a. photocatalyst
   b. photoinitiator
   c. photopolymerizer
   d. photo-oligomer
   _____

6. UV gels are typically not as _____ as monomer polymer enhancements.
   a. soft
   b. hard
   c. resilient
   d. easy to apply
   _____

7. When UV gel enhancements cure, they _____.
   a. harden to a solid material
   b. soften and remove easily
   c. become cooler
   d. become more viscous
   _____

8. A _____ resin is used for the one-color method of UV gel enhancement for clients who wish to wear colored polish or UV gel polish over the enhancement.
   a. white
   b. red
   c. pink
   d. clear
   _____

9. Which type of gel product is used to increase adhesion to the natural nail plate?
   a. UV building gel
   b. Pigmented UV gel
   c. UV bonding gel
   d. Self-leveling UV gel
   _____

10. Which type of UV gel is used to enhance the thickness of other gels while providing a smoother surface than some other UV building gels?
a. Self-leveling UV gel
b. Pigmented UV gel
c. UV gel polish
d. UV bonding gel

_____

11. UV building gels include any thick viscosity resin that allows the nail technician to build _____ to the fingernail.
a. bridge and curve
b. curve and mound
c. arch and slope
d. arch and curve

_____

12. UV gloss gels are also called sealing gels, finishing gels, or _____ gels.
a. buffing
b. patina
c. shine
d. luster

_____

13. Which type of UV gel does not produce an inhibition layer?
a. Traditional gloss gel
b. Tack-free gloss gel
c. Bonding gel
d. Self-leveling gel

_____

14. The tacky surface left on the nail after a UV gel has cured is known as the _____.
a. bonding seal
b. sealing bond
c. tack finish
d. inhibition layer

_____

15. What does nail primer do?
a. Properly cures the gel product
b. Improves adhesion of the gel product
c. Spreads the gel product
d. Secures the gel product

_____

16. It is recommended that you select a _____ abrasive for smoothing when performing UV gel services.
a. coarse
b. extra coarse
c. medium
d. fine

_____

17. If your client returns to the salon often with her enhancements broken, it is recommended that you try _____.
a. a UV gel with fiberglass
b. a self-leveling UV gel
c. a thicker UV gel
d. a thinner UV gel

_____

18. The special bulb that is used to cure UV gel nail enhancements is known as a _____ bulb.
a. halogen
b. soft white
c. UV or LED
d. fluorescent

_____

19. The specialized electronic device that powers and controls UV and LED bulbs to cure gel nail enhancements is known as a _____.
    a. UV bulb
    b. UV or LED lamp
    c. curing light unit
    d. electric light control   _____

20. Which of the following is a measurement of how much electricity is consumed by a UV lamp?
    a. Wattage
    b. Voltage
    c. Opacity
    d. Viscosity   _____

21. If UV bulbs are not changed regularly, service breakdown, skin irritation, and _____ are likely to occur.
    a. high electric bills
    b. irritating glare
    c. light dimming
    d. product sensitivity   _____

22. Which of the following is considered one of several standard UV bulbs?
    a. 60-watt
    b. 3-watt
    c. 9-watt
    d. 12-watt   _____

23. If you do not have the UV gel manufacturer's recommended cleanser, you should use _____ isopropanol or better.
    a. 80 percent
    b. 99 percent
    c. 75 percent
    d. 89 percent   _____

24. Gels commonly have _____ than monomer polymer nail enhancements.
    a. fewer colors
    b. more odors
    c. less odors
    d. less colors   _____

25. Gel polishes contain _____, cure under LED or UV light, and wear longer than traditional nail polish.
    a. less or no solvent
    b. less viscosity
    c. more solvent
    d. more viscosity   _____

26. Using the wrong LED light source on gel polish could drastically affect the _____.
    a. curing of the polish
    b. softening of the polish
    c. spreading of the polish
    d. durability of the polish   _____

27. Cured gel polish systems will _____ if the client hits her hands while the nail lacquer is still drying.
    a. spread evenly
    b. resist further drying
    c. not imprint or smudge
    d. not dry properly   _____

28. Soft UV gels are removed fairly easily with _____.
    a. polish remover
    b. acetone
    c. primer
    d. inhibitor   _____

29. When performing a one-color UV gel application on tips, use a _____ cleanser to remove oils from the fingernail prior to apply the tips.
    a. solvent-based
    b. solute
    c. acetone
    d. primer-based   _____

30. When performing a one-color UV gel application, it is recommended that the brush be _____ when applying the bonding or priming material.
    a. dry
    b. wet
    c. very wet
    d. slightly damp   _____

31. When applying UV gel, gently brush UV or LED gel onto the finger nail surface, including the free edge, leaving a _____ inch gap around the cuticle and sidewall area of the fingernail.
    a. 1/16
    b. 3/16
    c. 1/8
    d. 1/4   _____

32. Introducing air into the UV gel will reduce the strength of the cured gel and may lead to _____.
    a. lifting and splitting
    b. splitting and cracking
    c. bubbles and cracking
    d. lifting and falling off   _____

33. The nail plate will soften upon exposure to acetone and the scraping action could cause damage and alter the _____ of the fingernail.
    a. length
    b. strength
    c. shape
    d. color   _____

34. When performing a one-color UV gel application, after the first layer of gel has cured, it is recommended that you apply a small amount of _____.
    a. self-leveling UV gel
    b. UV building gel
    c. UV bonding gel
    d. UV gloss gel   _____

35. After filing a cured UV gel enhancement, it is recommended that you use a _____ to remove any dust and filings from the nail.
    a. disinfected sable brush
    b. disinfected nylon brush
    c. damp paper towel
    d. damp linen towel   _____

36. During a UV gel application, it is important to keep the brush and gel away from sunlight, UV gel lamps, and full-spectrum table lamps to prevent _____.
    a. overexposure of the fingers
    b. overexposure to heat
    c. overexposure to UV light
    d. premature hardening   ____

37. If the curve of the tip does not match the curve of the nail and the tip is spread _____, then the tips could crack lengthwise down the center.
    a. too wide   c. too thin
    b. a little wide   d. fully flat   ____

38. To create the smile line when performing a two-color UV gel application, you apply a coat of the white gel over the _____.
    a. tip and along   c. lunula and along the
       the sidewalls   sidewalls
    b. along the free   d. down the center
       edge   of the nail   ____

39. Compared to less opaque pigmented gels, more opaque pigmented gels typically _____.
    a. have the same viscosity   c. are thicker in viscosity
    b. have little viscosity   d. are thinner in viscosity   ____

40. When performing a two-color UV gel application, what is the next recommended step after removing the inhibition layer from the second layer of UV gel?
    a. Clean the fingernail
    b. Check the fingernail contours
    c. Apply nail oil
    d. Apply gloss UV gel   ____

41. When performing a UV gel application over forms, you will need UV gel, primer, brush, lamp, lint-free cleansing wipes, and _____.
    a. nippers   c. cleansing solution
    b. metal files   d. inhibitor   ____

42. When performing a UV gel maintenance service, after cleaning and dehydrating the fingernail, the next step is to _____.
    a. lightly buff the natural nail regrowth
    b. remove the dust from the nail surface
    c. lightly brush the gel on the nail
    d. cure the first UV gel   ____

43. When performing a UV gel polish application over a monomer and polymer enhancement, it is recommended that you use _____ when applying the first coat of gel polish.
    a. very little pressure
    b. ample pressure
    c. a dotting technique
    d. a circular technique
    _____

44. What is the recommended method for removing a soft UV gel application?
    a. Soaking nails in soak-off solution, then pushing it off with a wooden pusher
    b. Lightly buff the fingernail with a fine grit buffer
    c. Clean the nail enhancements with a nail brush
    d. Soak nail in warm water, then pry off with nippers
    _____

CHAPTER 19: THE CREATIVE TOUCH

1. Ways to create client interest in nail art include displaying artful tips in a glass case or frame, inserting photos of creative nail art into a portfolio, and _____.
   a. showing written testimonies from clients
   b. wearing beautiful nail art on your own nails
   c. posting a list of client contact information who have nail art
   d. display only one medium and prepare to discuss others ____

2. Nail art should be priced based on the cost of materials, time investment, the nail technician's level of expertise, the clientele, and _____.
   a. the area
   b. the salon's budget
   c. salon decor
   d. your financial needs ____

3. The light we see reflected from a surface is called _____.
   a. ultraviolet light
   b. infrared light
   c. chromatics
   d. color ____

4. Nail polish looks _____ when all colors are reflected.
   a. black
   b. white
   c. red
   d. blue ____

5. Which of the following is *not* a primary color?
   a. Red
   b. Green
   c. Yellow
   d. Blue ____

6. When you mix equal parts of two primary colors, you create _____.
   a. a secondary color
   b. a tertiary color
   c. a complementary color
   d. an intermediate color ____

7. The colors directly resulting from mixing equal parts of one primary color and one of its nearest secondary colors are called _____.
   a. pastel colors
   b. analogous colors
   c. complementary colors
   d. tertiary colors ____

8. Which of the following is *not* a secondary color?
   a. Orange
   b. Yellow
   c. Green
   d. Violet ____

9. Tertiary colors are also known as _____.
   a. secondary colors
   b. analogous colors
   c. intermediate colors
   d. complementary colors ____

10. When complementary colors are applied side by side, they _____ each other, making each other stand out or *pop*.
   a. enhance
   b. stabilize
   c. neutralize
   d. minimize
   _____

11. Colors located beside each other on the color wheel are known as _____.
   a. intermediate colors
   b. tertiary colors
   c. complementary colors
   d. analogous colors
   _____

12. Red-violet and blue-green are examples of _____ colors.
   a. secondary
   b. tertiary
   c. complementary
   d. analogous
   _____

13. For a traditional French manicure look, the nail bed (up to the free edge) is one color, such as pink, peach, or _____, and the free edge of the nail plate is another color such as white.
   a. blue
   b. green
   c. beige
   d. aqua
   _____

14. Which term refers to a swirled effect created when you combine two or more colors while wet, and then mix them on the nail?
   a. Marbleizing
   b. Color blocking
   c. French manicure
   d. Color fading
   _____

15. When the top of a client's nail is light pink, the bottom is dark pink, and the middle is a combination of the two colors, this is known as _____.
   a. color blocking
   b. color fading
   c. marbleizing
   d. swirling
   _____

16. The tool used to create the marbleizing effect is called a _____.
   a. style brush
   b. polish pen
   c. pusher
   d. stylus
   _____

17. In a French manicure, the curved line where the pink and the white color meet on the nail is called _____.
   a. color differentiator
   b. color separator
   c. the smile line
   d. the smile curve
   _____

18. The very end of the bristles on a brush, farthest away from the handle, is referred to as the _____ depending on the style of the brush.
    a. tip or chisel edge   c. ferrule or flat edge
    b. belly or round edge   d. heel or box edge   _____

19. A nail technician should master the _____ technique and variations of it to stay competitive in the marketplace.
    a. gold leafing   c. free-hand painting
    b. French manicure   d. air brushing   _____

20. The metal band around the brush that helps to hold the bristles in place is called _____.
    a. a mandrel   c. a ferrule
    b. the heel   d. the banding   _____

21. The area in which the bristles meet the ferrule is called the _____ of the brush.
    a. belly   c. tip
    b. crust   d. heel   _____

22. A liner brush is not specifically recommended for_____.
    a. line work   c. blending
    b. outlining   d. lettering   _____

23. A _____ brush has a square tip with long bristles.
    a. liner   c. round
    b. flat   d. spotter   _____

24. A spotter brush is also commonly known as a _____ brush.
    a. detailer   c. fan
    b. striper   d. round   _____

25. Which term refers to the amount of force that an artist applies to the brush while stroking?
    a. Pull   c. Position
    b. Pressure   d. Push   _____

26. Which term refers to how you hold the brush on the nail?
    a. Pressure   c. Push
    b. Pull   d. Position   _____

27. Which of the following is not an example of a versatile design stroke?
    a. Comma   c. Branch
    b. Ribbon   d. Teardrop   _____

28. When applying 3-D art over nail polish, ensure the polish
    is _____ before continuing.
    a. completely cured   c. partially dry
    b. completely dry   d. pliable   _____

29. The more paint you put on the very tip of the brush,
    the _____ the beginning of the stroke will be.
    a. wider   c. narrower
    b. deeper   d. thinner   _____

30. Any element that can be applied to the nail as art is
    considered _____.
    a. an adhesive   c. a decal
    b. adornment   d. an embellishment   _____

31. A nail art element that does not have its own adhesive
    backing, you can adhere it with resin, tip adhesive,
    or _____.
    a. tape   c. paste
    b. base coat   d. top coat   _____

32. The ideal airbrush systems for nail art are designed
    for _____ paint.
    a. high-gloss   c. gravity-fed
    b. fast-drying   d. semi-gloss   _____

33. Which of the following is not part of the handle of an
    airbrush machine?
    a. Trigger   c. Needle
    b. Fluid nozzle   d. Compressor   _____

34. The _____ connects the handle of an airbrush
    machine to the compressor.
    a. air hose   c. release line
    b. cap   d. pressure regulator   _____

35. When using an airbrush machine, most nail professionals
    work at a pressure between _____.
    a. 45 and 55 psi   c. 15 and 20 psi
    b. 85 and 100 psi   d. 25 and 35 psi   _____

36. When applied correctly, airbrush paint appears _____.
    a. bright and powdery   c. bright and glossy
    b. dull and powdery   d. dull and glossy   _____

37. To create designs or specific shapes when airbrushing, you can use _____, a thin plastic with a sticky back that is cut by a machine into various shapes.
   a. a model
   b. a precut diagram
   c. an airbrush stencil
   d. a blueprint
   _____

38. When preparing for a nail competition, it is recommended that you first _____.
   a. sketch out your idea
   b. determine what the theme is
   c. practice with a model
   d. put together your competition kit
   _____

39. During the _____, the competition director or head judge will review the rules and guidelines to ensure everyone understands them and is able to comply.
   a. briefing
   b. judging
   c. application period
   d. intermission
   _____

40. The _____ category includes all freehand painting techniques that are not raised.
   a. flat art
   b. 3-D art
   c. fantasy art
   d. design sculpture
   _____

41. Any art that protrudes from the nail falls into the _____ nail art category.
   a. fantasy
   b. design sculpture
   c. embellishment
   d. 3-D
   _____

42. The term _____ is a description used for nail art when more than one nail art medium is used to create a design.
   a. "flat art"
   b. "3-D art"
   c. "mixed-media"
   d. "freestyle art"
   _____

43. In _____ competitions, the technician is limited only by his or her own imagination.
   a. Grand Illusion
   b. Fantasy Art
   c. Fanciful
   d. Dream Vision
   _____

44. You will not need which of the following items when creating crystal art on polish using embellishments?
   a. Nail forms
   b. Top coat
   c. Tweezers
   d. Brush-on adhesive
   _____

45. When creating crystal art on polish using embellishments, it is recommended that you _____ first.
   a. place smaller crystals
   b. apply a base coat
   c. place larger crystals
   d. allow adhesive to dry
   _____

CHAPTER 20: SEEKING EMPLOYMENT

1. Before you can obtain a position as a nail technician you must first pass your regulatory agency's licensing examination and _____.
   a. secure the required credentials from the applicable regulatory agency
   b. network with industry professionals to determine job opportunities
   c. schedule and complete at least six employment interviews
   d. prepare a complete resume and employment portfolio   ____

2. Factors that will affect how well you perform during the licensing examination include your physical and psychological state, your memory, time management, and your _____.
   a. stamina   c. academic skills
   b. awareness   d. social skills   ____

3. A test-wise student is one who understands _____.
   a. the importance of doing well in school
   b. the strategies for successfully taking tests
   c. the importance of attitude
   d. that going the extra mile makes a difference   ____

4. The word *holistic* refers to _____.
   a. the whole you   c. a complete scholastic experience
   b. the whole test   d. an integrated education   ____

5. An important part of preparing for your licensing exam is maintaining good physical, emotional, and spiritual health, including _____.
   a. sharp personal habits
   b. projecting a positive attitude
   c. excellent personal hygiene
   d. sound diet and eating habits   ____

6. On the day of the test, it is not recommended that you _____.
   a. relax and try to slow down physically
   b. review the material lightly on the day of the exam
   c. avoid monitoring the time to reduce your stress
   d. arrive early with a self-confident attitude   ____

7. The process of reaching logical conclusions by employing logical reasoning is known as _____.
   a. deductive reasoning
   b. conclusive reasoning
   c. presumptive reasoning
   d. deductive justification _____

8. In test questions, the basic question or problem is known as _____.
   a. a query
   b. the stem
   c. a conundrum
   d. the root _____

9. Which of the following is an example of an absolute?
   a. Some
   b. Never
   c. Usually
   d. Little _____

10. When two choices in a multiple-choice question are similar _____.
    a. one is always right
    b. both are usually right
    c. both are usually wrong
    d. one is probably right _____

11. To better prepare for the practical portion of the examination, you should practice the correct skills required in the test frequently and _____.
    a. participate in mock licensing examinations
    b. take as many tools and implements as you can fit in the kit bag
    c. be concerned about the behavior of other test candidates
    d. dress casually and wear athletic shoes _____

12. Which of the following is not a characteristic that will help you get the position you want and help you keep it?
    a. Apathy
    b. Strong work ethic
    c. Good technical skills
    d. Self-motivation _____

13. When you have _____, you are committed to a strong code of moral and artistic values.
    a. integrity
    b. motivation
    c. enthusiasm
    d. curiosity _____

14. Having _____ means taking pride in your work and committing yourself to consistently performing a good job for your clients, employer, and salon team.
    a. professional integrity
    b. a strong work ethic
    c. strong technical skills
    d. exceptional enthusiasm _____

15. There are nearly _____ professional salons in the United States.
    a. 313,000
    b. 370,000
    c. 1.6 million
    d. 97,000 _____

16. The average independent salon may have as many as
    _____ nail technicians working there regularly.
    a. 5   c. 15
    b. 10   d. 20   ____

17. The majority of professional nail salons and spas are

    _____.
    a. large corporate salon chains
    b. independent salon chains
    c. franchises
    d. small independent salons   ____

18. Independent salon chains usually have _____ or
    more salons that are owned by one individual or two or more
    partners.
    a. 2   c. 5
    b. 4   d. 10   ____

19. With large national salon chains, decisions regarding size,
    decor, hours, services, prices, advertising, and _____
    are made at the corporate headquarters.
    a. profit targets   c. licensing requirements
    b. license fees   d. esthetician scheduling   ____

20. Basic value-priced operations generally _____.
    a. pay nail technicians by the hour
    b. hire highly seasoned technicians
    c. depend primarily on an established client base
    d. usually charge $30 or more for manicures   ____

21. High-end salons or day spas hire practitioners whose
    technical expertise, personal appearance, and _____
    meet their high standards.
    a. social skills   c. personal goals
    b. communication skills   d. personal beliefs   ____

22. Resume preparation guidelines include keeping it simple,
    limiting it to one page, and including _____.
    a. a personal photo
    b. personal references
    c. a cover letter
    d. a list of personal hobbies   ____

23. A written summary of a person's education and work
    experience is known as _____.
    a. a resume   c. a portfolio
    b. a synopsis   d. an encapsulation   ____

24. On average, a potential employer will scan your resume for about _____ before deciding whether to grant you an interview.
    a. 20 seconds
    c. 60 seconds
    b. 45 seconds
    d. 2 minutes _____

25. Accomplishment statements highlight your basic duties and responsibilities and the best way to show concrete accomplishments is to include _____.
    a. a list of achievements
    c. numbers or percentages
    b. income and expense ratios
    d. glowing words and adjectives _____

26. There is no better time for you to achieve significant accomplishments for your resume than _____.
    a. while you are in school
    c. during high school
    b. during your first job
    d. while growing up _____

27. Make your resume easy to read by using concise, clear sentences and avoid overwriting _____.
    a. and overstating goals
    c. and making it too brief
    b. and flowery language
    d. and making it too easy to read _____

28. Skills that you have mastered in other jobs that can be put to use in a new position are called _____.
    a. transportable skills
    c. transferable skills
    b. transmittable skills
    d. deliverable skills _____

29. A collection, usually bound, of photos and documents that reflect your skills, accomplishments, and abilities in a chosen career field is called _____.
    a. a professional resume
    c. a career synopsis
    b. an employment binder
    d. an employment portfolio _____

30. One of the most important steps in the process of job hunting is determining what you want in a salon or spa environment and narrowing your search so you can _____.
    a. target potential coworkers
    b. find the best parking areas
    c. find the neighborhood of choice
    d. target potential employers _____

31. Connecting with people, communities, and local businesses to build mutually beneficial relationships is known as _____.
    a. socializing
    c. information exchanging
    b. networking
    d. connecting _____

122

32. When you visit a salon for networking purposes, using a checklist and keeping it on file for future reference is helpful in making informed _____.
    a. interview decisions
    b. networking decisions
    c. comparisons between establishments
    d. socializing decisions   ____

33. After visiting a salon, it is recommended that you always _____.
    a. return for a second visit
    b. critique the salon to the manager
    c. ask for an interview
    d. send a thank you note   ____

34. When you go to a job interview, the documents you bring with you should include the contact information of former employers, the contact information of your nearest relative not living with you, your social security number, and _____.
    a. your driver's license number
    b. your license plate number
    c. your preferred work hours
    d. your best handbag or wallet   ____

35. It is recommended that you obtain how many interview outfits?
    a. One or two   c. No fewer than three
    b. No more than one   d. At least five   ____

36. The accessories you wear with your interview outfit should be fashionable and _____.
    a. busy   c. large
    b. functional   d. expensive   ____

37. When you go to a job interview, it is recommended that you take your resume, your portfolio, and _____.
    a. important facts and figures
    b. your postsecondary school transcript
    c. your high school transcript
    d. your prior year income tax statement   ____

38. Which of the following is not a typical question asked by a potential employer?
    a. Can you assume management responsibilities immediately?
    b. What skills do you feel are your strongest?
    c. What are your career goals?
    d. What days and hours are you available for work?   ____

39. On the day of the interview, it is recommended that you arrive early, smile, use good posture, be polite and courteous, and _____.
    a. refer to your cell phone often
    b. speak clearly to be understood
    c. chew gum and smoke if it is offered
    d. constructively criticize former employers ____

40. It is permissible to ask the age of an applicant younger than _____.
    a. 18   c. 30
    b. 21   d. 65   ____

41. An employer is allowed to ask whether you _____.
    a. are a U.S. citizen   c. have disabilities
    b. use drugs or tobacco   d. have medical problems   ____

42. Employers can legally require you to sign an employment contract, which usually includes a noncompete clause and a _____.
    a. schedule commitment
    b. continuing education requirement
    c. salary/pay restriction
    d. confidentiality agreement ____

43. In preparing your portfolio and writing about why you chose a career in nail technology, you may wish to include a description of your philosophy about the importance of teamwork and _____.
    a. self-sufficiency
    b. your independence
    c. your role as a team member
    d. your ability to work independently ____

44. When taking a multiple choice text, it is important to _____.
    a. scan the questions quickly before answering
    b. read the entire question carefully, including all the choices
    c. ignore obviously incorrect answers
    d. ignore absolutes in the various answers ____

45. What is the appropriate time period to wait before calling a salon after sending your resume and cover letter?
    a. One day   c. Two weeks
    b. One week   d. One month   ____

CHAPTER 21: ON THE JOB

1. It is recommended that while you network with mentors, nail professionals, educators, and classmates, you ask questions, take advice, _____, and consider all your options.
    a. talk about your skills
    b. talk your successes
    c. talk about your goals
    d. listen to their comments ____

2. In a service business such as nail technology, your work primarily revolves around _____.
    a. making yourself happy
    b. serving your clients
    c. scheduling your clients
    d. interacting with coworkers ____

3. As you serve your clients, important behaviors include putting others first, being true to your word, _____, being a problem solver, and being courteous.
    a. being tardy only rarely
    b. turning problems over to others
    c. being punctual
    d. putting yourself first ____

4. Getting to work on time shows respect not only for your clients, but also for _____.
    a. yourself
    b. your family
    c. your friends
    d. your coworkers ____

5. In a professional environment, it is important to always perform quality work, meet the clients' expectations, and be well versed in _____.
    a. the latest nail trends
    b. recent headline news
    c. current political affairs
    d. the latest fashion trends ____

6. You can remain knowledgeable about the changes in the industry by reading industry magazines, attending trade shows and networking events, and _____.
    a. reading local newspapers
    b. attending classes
    c. observing coworker techniques
    d. attending community events ____

7. Being a team player means following several workplace principles including being concerned with the success of others, being willing to help, _____, and remaining positive.
    a. working only with good friends
    b. sharing information about clients
    c. keeping best practices to yourself
    d. sharing your knowledge with coworkers ____

8. Salon management should be loyal to the clients and
   _____.
   a. the area businesses   c. their staff
   b. themselves   d. their vendors   _____

9. A document that outlines all the duties and responsibilities of
   a particular position in the salon or spa is called _____.
   a. a duty description   c. a job description
   b. a duty outline   d. a responsibility report   _____

10. A key element in conflict resolution is _____.
    a. addressing the situation publicly
    b. being accountable for your part in the situation
    c. placing blame where it belongs
    d. explaining why your point of view is correct   _____

11. If you are unclear about something listed as your
    responsibility, it is up to you to _____.
    a. rationalize its meaning
    b. ask for clarification
    c. change it to your philosophy
    d. fulfill it to the best of your ability   _____

12. When you accept a salon position, what you will be paid for
    your work is called _____.
    a. compensation   c. dispensation
    b. remuneration   d. payment   _____

13. Which of the following is not a standard method of
    compensation in the nail industry?
    a. Straight salary   c. Tips only
    b. Commission percentage   d. Salary plus commission   _____

14. If you don't think you can make enough money solely on a
    commission basis, then take a position in a salon or spa that
    will pay you an hourly wage until you _____.
    a. can reduce your living expenses
    b. build your clientele
    c. can get a second job
    d. increase salon service pricing   _____

15. Customers who are loyal to a particular nail technician are
    known as your _____.
    a. regular patrons   c. client base
    b. client list   d. career partners   _____

16. If you are offered a set salary each week, in lieu of an hourly rate, that salary must _____.
    a. be equal to the minimum wage for the number of hours you work
    b. include overtime for hours worked over 30
    c. include overtime pay for management positions
    d. not include overtime pay for hours over 40 _____

17. The commission paid to a nail technician working on a commission-only basis generally ranges from _____.
    a. 5–20 percent   c. 15–30 percent
    b. 75–90 percent   d. 25–60 percent _____

18. If you work under a commission payment structure, the salon usually provides the _____ you will need to perform nail services.
    a. nail brushes   c. electric drills
    b. products   d. files _____

19. Nail technicians can increase their chances of building a solid and loyal clientele more quickly if they live in an area with lots of potential clients, have advanced training, skills, certifications, artistic abilities, and _____.
    a. live in a highly competitive and saturated market
    b. provide only a select few services
    c. limit work hours to those usually busy
    d. employ marketing and publicity strategies _____

20. A _____ payment structure is often used to motivate nail technicians to perform more services.
    a. tips-only   c. salary-plus-commission
    b. salary-only   d. salary-minus-commission _____

21. Tips are income in addition to regular compensation and must be tracked and _____.
    a. kept in a safe place   c. received with grace
    b. shared with coworkers d. reported as regular income _____

22. How often must tips be recorded?
    a. Daily   c. Weekly
    b. Monthly   d. Never _____

23. The best way to keep tabs on your progress is to ask for feedback from your clients, salon or spa manager, and _____.
    a. friends   c. family
    b. neighbors   d. key coworkers _____

24. Evaluations are commonly scheduled 90 days after hiring and then _____ after that.
    a. three times a year
    c. once a year
    b. twice a year
    d. every two years
    _____

25. Ask a _____ to sit in on one of your consultations and make note of areas where you can improve.
    a. senior nail technician
    c. junior nail technician
    b. loyal client
    d. loyal friend
    _____

26. Not paying back your student loan or other type of mortgage is known as defaulting, and it can have serious consequences regarding your personal and professional _____.
    a. credit
    c. relationships
    b. reputation
    d. budget
    _____

27. If you know you will need to take home $3,000 per month to support your needs, you will want to calculate how this translates into the _____.
    a. number of hours you work
    b. number of clients in your client base
    c. number of days you work
    d. number of clients and services you perform per month
    _____

28. One recommended method for increasing your disposable income is _____.
    a. to spend more money
    c. to reduce service prices
    b. to perform fewer services
    d. to spend less money
    _____

29. If you have a loyal client base and a mastery of services offered, it is appropriate to increase your prices _____ by a reasonable amount.
    a. every week
    c. every month
    b. every quarter
    d. every year or two
    _____

30. It is recommended that you speak with _____ for advice on how to reduce your credit card debt, invest your money, and plan for retirement.
    a. an attorney
    c. a financial planner
    b. a marketing expert
    d. an accountant
    _____

31. The practice of recommending and selling additional services to clients that you may perform is known as _____.
    a. ticket upgrading
    c. retailing
    b. prescribing
    d. wholesaling
    _____

32. The act of recommending and selling quality products to clients for at-home nail care is called _____.
   a. wholesaling
   b. retailing
   c. ticket upgrading
   d. prescribing
   _____

33. To be successful in sales, you need _____, determination, and a good personality.
   a. timidity
   b. firmness
   c. assertiveness
   d. ambition
   _____

34. Recognizing the client's needs and _____ lays the foundation for successful selling.
   a. personality
   b. preferences
   c. budget
   d. ego
   _____

35. You become _____ by knowing about the products you are selling and by believing that they are as good as you say.
   a. confident
   b. reluctant
   c. timid
   d. assertive
   _____

36. What is the standard retail sales commission for nail technicians?
   a. 5 percent
   b. 10 percent
   c. 15 percent
   d. 20 percent
   _____

37. One way that is recommended to get the conversation started about retailing products is that you _____.
   a. keep products stored neatly in a closed cabinet
   b. discuss the procedure you are following during the service
   c. place products in the clients' hands whenever possible
   d. keep retail areas simple and subdued
   _____

38. If you are going to send a client a birthday card with a special offer, it is recommended that you send it out _____.
   a. the week before the client's birthday
   b. about one month before the client's birthday
   c. on the client's birthday
   d. a few days before the client's birthday
   _____

39. If you send a client a birthday card with a special offer, it is recommended that the offer be valid _____.
   a. with no expiration date
   b. for the rest of the year
   c. only on the client's birthday
   d. only during the birthday month
   _____

40. You can expand your client base by being reliable, respectful, positive, and _____.
    a. professional
    b. assertive
    c. approachable
    d. amateurish

    _____

41. Your responsibility is to be the client's _____.
    a. psychiatrist
    b. relationship counselor
    c. nail technician
    d. friend

    _____

42. When selling, it is recommended that after you establish rapport with the client, you _____.
    a. recommend products or services
    b. determine the client's needs
    c. emphasize product benefits
    d. close the sale

    _____

43. It is recommended that you rebook a client _____.
    a. before she leaves the salon
    b. before she arrives at the salon
    c. while providing services
    d. after she leaves the salon

    _____

44. How long should a client be in the salon?
    a. As long as you can keep him or her there comfortably
    b. As long as it takes to adequately complete the service
    c. As long as the conversation remains interesting
    d. As little time as possible

    _____

45. After researching web articles regarding building a client base, make a list of the suggestions that seem suitable and try one every _____.
    a. day or two
    b. week or two
    c. two or three months
    d. quarter

    _____

CHAPTER 22: THE SALON BUSINESS

1. Booth rental, also known as _____ rental, is when a nail technician rents a booth in a salon or spa.
   a. station
   b. space
   c. chair
   d. leasing ____

2. In a booth rental arrangement, a nail technician generally is solely responsible for her own clientele, furniture, telephone, advertising, towels, insurance, laundry, supplies, and _____.
   a. signs on the building
   b. record keeping and accounting
   c. utility bills
   d. providing parking for clients ____

3. The state board in _____ does not recognize booth rental as an acceptable method of doing business.
   a. Pennsylvania
   b. New Mexico
   c. South Dakota
   d. Tennessee ____

4. Opening your own salon or spa is a huge undertaking, financially, physically, and _____, because you will face challenges that are complex and unfamiliar to you.
   a. socially
   b. internally
   c. personally
   d. mentally ____

5. A _____ statement is a long-term picture of what a business is to become and what it will look like when it gets there.
   a. mission
   b. vision
   c. production
   d. projection ____

6. Which term refers to a set of benchmarks that, once achieved, help you to realize your mission and your vision?
   a. Proprietors
   b. Business plan
   c. Goals
   d. Capital ____

7. In your business timeline, the time to tend to the business, its clientele, and its employees and to grow and expand the business so that it is profitable, is in years _____.
   a. 2–5
   b. 5–7
   c. 7–9
   d. 11–20 ____

8. In determining the feasibility of your business, you must address if you have _____ that will set your business apart from other nail businesses in your area.
   a. a dream or goal
   b. a special skill or talent
   c. a color scheme and decor
   d. a salon or spa theme ____

9. A business that is owned and operated by one person, although the owner may have employees, is called _____.
   a. a corporation
   b. an S corporation
   c. an LLC
   d. a sole proprietorship ____

10. In a sole proprietorship, the owner determines the policies and has the last say in decision making as well as _____.
    a. assuming expenses, receiving profits, and bearing all losses
    b. having protection of his or her personal assets
    c. having less tax liability than a corporation
    d. the ability to raise capital more easily than a corporation ____

11. A business structure in which two or more people share ownership, although not necessarily equally, is called _____.
    a. a corporation
    b. an LLC
    c. a sole proprietorship
    d. a partnership ____

12. People often enter into a partnership arrangement to have more capital or money to invest in a business and to _____.
    a. have less debt liability
    b. have more responsibility
    c. have help operating the business
    d. have more independent decision making ____

13. A corporation is an ownership structure controlled by one or more stockholders and is one of the best ways to _____.
    a. organize hidden assets
    b. protect personal assets
    c. have a more rigid business operation
    d. have less transparency to the public ____

14. Who owns a corporation?
    a. The stockholders
    b. The board of directors
    c. The chairperson of the board
    d. The president of the company ____

15. Employees of a corporation pay income tax on _____.
    a. the corporate profits   c. monthly benefits
    b. the salary that is drawn   d. earnings distributions   _____

16. When opening your own business, it is recommended that
    you consult with _____ to find out the ways in which
    your business may be registered for tax purposes.
    a. an attorney and accountant c. a financial advisor
    b. a stockbroker   d. a shareholder   _____

17. To become an S corporation, the S corporation status is
    elected through _____.
    a. the IRS
    b. the state corporation commission
    c. the state insurance commission
    d. the state regulatory agency   _____

18. What does LLC stand for?
    a. Legal Liability Company   c. Limited Liability
                                      Corporation
    b. Legal Liability Corporation d. Limited Liability Company   _____

19. A _____ is a written plan of a business as it is seen in
    the present and envisioned in the future, to follow throughout
    the entire process of starting your own business.
    a. vision statement   c. business plan
    b. mission statement   d. financial statement   _____

20. Which part of a business plan describes how the business
    will run administratively?
    a. Organizational plan   c. Executive summary
    b. Vision statement   d. Salon policies   _____

21. Which part of the business plan outlines all of the research
    obtained regarding the clients your business will target and
    their needs, wants, and habits?
    a. Organizational plan   c. Supporting documents
    b. Marketing plan   d. Financial documents   _____

22. Before purchasing an existing nail salon, _____ to
    determine the actual value of the business once current
    owner's bookings are taken out of the equation.
    a. seek professional assistance
    b. determine retail sales
    c. look over the appointment book
    d. conduct a financial audit   _____

23. It is important to protect your business by installing adequate locks, a fire alarm system, and _____.
    a. a burglar alarm system c. a life alert system
    b. a new ventilation system d. a carbon monoxide alert _____

24. If you sell retail, you may need to obtain _____ or other license.
    a. a business certificate c. a seller's permit
    b. a retail registration d. an inventory control permit _____

25. Information about a specific population, including data on race, age, income, and educational attainment is known as _____.
    a. human characteristics c. area census
    b. demographics d. governmental statistics _____

26. The ongoing, reoccurring processes or activities involved in the running of a business for the purpose of producing income and value is known as _____.
    a. standard activities c. salon operations
    b. standard procedures d. operating policies _____

27. A typical salon spends about _____ of its total gross income on rent.
    a. 3 percent c. 13 percent
    b. 5 percent d. 53 percent _____

28. Which of the following expenses typically represents about 3 percent of a salon's total gross income?
    a. Depreciation c. Utilities
    b. Cleaning d. Insurance _____

29. A typical salon spends about 1.5 percent of its total gross income on which of the following expenses?
    a. Telephone c. Advertising
    b. Repairs d. Supplies _____

30. About _____ of a typical salon's total gross income is profit.
    a. 53 percent c. 5 percent
    b. 85 percent d. 15 percent _____

31. A _____ is someone who is trained to do everything from recording sales and doing payroll to generating a profit-and-loss statement.
    a. receptionist
    b. full-charge bookkeeper
    c. tax attorney
    d. payroll service representative _____

32. Supplies that are sold to clients are called _____.
    a. consumption supplies   c. reduction supplies
    b. wholesale supplies   d. retail supplies _____

33. Service records should include the contact information, the products used, and _____ for each client.
    a. personality type
    b. the service results obtained
    c. fashion personality style
    d. the amount of time the client was in salon _____

34. When renovating a salon, it is recommended that you consult with _____.
    a. a professional equipment and furniture supplier
    b. a professional design attorney
    c. a professional salon architect
    d. a professional salon trainer _____

35. Which of the following is not an important consideration when interviewing potential employees?
    a. Their personal grooming   c. Their age
    b. Their communication skills d. Their overall attitude _____

36. Which part of the salon is considered the salon's nerve center?
    a. The manager's office   c. The dispensary
    b. The reception area   d. The nail station _____

37. The reception area should be well stocked with _____.
    a. consumption supplies   c. business cards
    b. terrycloth towels   d. reference materials _____

38. During slow periods, it is customary for the receptionist to perform other duties such as straightening up the reception area, maintaining inventory, and _____.
    a. completing daily reports
    b. updating employee records
    c. cleaning the dispensary
    d. redesigning business cards _____

39. Which of the following is not a common responsibility of a salon receptionist?
   a. Preparing the daily appointment information
   b. Recommending other services to the client
   c. Answering the phone
   d. Performing employee evaluations ___

40. The receptionist must have an appearance that conveys the salon's image, knowledge of the various services offered, and _____.
   a. unlimited patience   c. a reserved personality
   b. unlimited resources   d. a stoic demeanor ___

41. When using the telephone, you should use a pleasant voice, speak clearly, use correct grammar, and _____.
   a. express impatience
   b. be concise and to the point
   c. show interest and concern
   d. take other calls while the first call is on hold ___

42. When answering the phone, it is important to _____.
   a. answer promptly
   b. turn on a voicemail message
   c. answer within five rings
   d. talk with a salon client while answering ___

43. If a client calls to make an appointment with her favorite nail technician at a certain time, and the nail technician is not available, the receptionist should first _____.
   a. refer the client to another salon
   b. suggest other available times
   c. offer to put the client on a waiting list
   d. suggest another nail technician in the salon ___

44. What is considered the best form of advertising?
   a. Business cards   c. Yellow page advertising
   b. Satisfied clients   d. Television advertising ___

45. In considering the general reasons people buy products, we can assume that people are motivated to _____.
   a. fill an urge   c. satisfy a need
   b. have the best of everything   d. impulse purchase ___

Part II: Answers to Exam Review for Nail Technology

CHAPTER 1: HISTORY AND CAREER OPPORTUNITIES

ANSWER KEY AND CORE BOOK PAGE REFERENCES

QUESTION	PAGE	QUESTION	PAGE
1. b	4	24. a	7
2. c	7	25. c	7
3. a	5	26. d	7
4. c	5	27. a	7
5. b	5	28. b	7
6. a	5	29. c	7
7. c	5	30. b	7
8. a	5	31. a	8
9. b	5	32. c	8
10. a	5	33. d	8
11. b	5	34. a	7
12. a	5	35. c	7
13. c	5	36. b	8
14. d	5	37. c	7
15. c	5	38. d	7
16. d	6	39. d	8
17. d	6	40. b	9
18. b	6	41. c	9
19. b	6	42. d	9
20. c	6	43. b	10
21. a	6	44. d	10
22. b	6	45. a	9
23. d	7		

CHAPTER 2: LIFE SKILLS

ANSWER KEY AND CORE BOOK PAGE REFERENCES

QUESTION	PAGE	QUESTION	PAGE
1. c	15	12. d	17
2. d	15	13. a	19
3. a	15	14. c	20
4. b	16	15. b	20
5. c	16	16. b	20
6. a	16	17. b	20
7. d	17	18. a	20
8. c	16	19. d	21
9. b	16	20. b	26
10. d	17	21. c	21
11. b	17	22. a	21

QUESTION	PAGE	QUESTION	PAGE
23. b	21	35. d	26
24. a	23	36. c	27–28
25. d	23	37. a	26
26. d	24	38. b	27
27. c	24	39. c	27
28. b	24	40. a	28
29. a	25	41. c	27
30. d	25	42. c	28
31. b	26	43. b	28
32. c	26	44. b	28
33. a	26	45. a	28
34. b	26		

CHAPTER 3: YOUR PROFESSIONAL IMAGE

ANSWER KEY AND CORE BOOK PAGE REFERENCES

QUESTION	PAGE	QUESTION	PAGE
1. b	33	24. b	35
2. d	33	25. d	36
3. a	33	26. d	36
4. c	33	27. c	36
5. a	33	28. a	37
6. a	33	29. b	37
7. c	33	30. c	37
8. d	33	31. d	37
9. b	34	32. b	34
10. d	34	33. d	37
11. a	34	34. a	37
12. c	34	35. c	37
13. a	34	36. b	37
14. c	38	37. d	37
15. b	34	38. c	37
16. a	34	39. c	38
17. c	34	40. a	38
18. d	35	41. a	38
19. b	34	42. a	38
20. a	34	43. c	37
21. d	35	44. b	36
22. c	35	45. b	33
23. a	35		

CHAPTER 4: COMMUNICATING FOR SUCCESS

ANSWER KEY AND CORE BOOK PAGE REFERENCES

QUESTION	PAGE	QUESTION	PAGE
1. d	42	3. c	43
2. a	43	4. b	44

5. a	44	26. c	52
6. d	45	27. b	52
7. c	45	28. a	53
8. c	45	29. a	53
9. a	49	30. d	54
10. b	49	31. d	43
11. d	45	32. b	45
12. a	46–47	33. c	56
13. b	45	34. d	55
14. c	48	35. a	56
15. a	48	36. c	57
16. a	48	37. b	57
17. c	50	38. a	57
18. a	49	39. c	57
19. c	49	40. c	57
20. a	50	41. a	43
21. c	50	42. d	44
22. d	50	43. c	45
23. b	52	44. a	45
24. a	52	45. a	48
25. d	52		

CHAPTER 5: INFECTION CONTROL: PRINCIPLES AND PRACTICES

ANSWER KEY AND CORE BOOK PAGE REFERENCES

QUESTION	PAGE	QUESTION	PAGE
1. c	62	21. c	67
2. a	62	22. b	67
3. b	62	23. d	67
4. d	63	24. c	68
5. c	63	25. c	69
6. b	63	26. d	69
7. a	63	27. a	69
8. c	63	28. b	70
9. d	63	29. d	70
10. b	64	30. d	70
11. a	64	31. b	70
12. b	64	32. a	71
13. c	64	33. d	71
14. a	65	34. b	72
15. d	65	35. c	73
16. b	65	36. b	74
17. b	66	37. c	74
18. c	66	38. d	74
19. d	67	39. a	75
20. a	67	40. c	75

41. a	76	50. d	82
42. c	76	51. c	83
43. d	76	52. a	84
44. c	77	53. b	84
45. c	79	54. d	86
46. c	80	55. c	85
47. a	80	56. a	86
48. b	80	57. d	90
49. a	81		

CHAPTER 6: GENERAL ANATOMY AND PHYSIOLOGY

ANSWER KEY AND CORE BOOK PAGE REFERENCES

QUESTION	PAGE	QUESTION	PAGE
1. b	105	26. b	114
2. a	105	27. c	114
3. b	105	28. a	115
4. d	105–106	29. b	115
5. b	106	30. a	116
6. c	107	31. c	116
7. a	107	32. d	116
8. d	107	33. c	116
9. a	108	34. b	117
10. b	109	35. d	118
11. c	109	36. a	118
12. a	109	37. a	118
13. d	109	38. c	118
14. b	109	39. b	119
15. a	110	40. d	119
16. b	110	41. b	119
17. b	111	42. c	120
18. c	111	43. c	120
19. a	111	44. a	120
20. d	111	45. b	120
21. a	112	46. d	120
22. b	112	47. c	120
23. a	113	48. c	122
24. c	113	49. b	123
25. b	114	50. a	124

CHAPTER 7: SKIN STRUCTURE, GROWTH, AND NUTRITION

ANSWER KEY AND CORE BOOK PAGE REFERENCES

QUESTION	PAGE	QUESTION	PAGE
1. b	128	4. a	129
2. c	128	5. c	129
3. b	128	6. d	129

7. c	129	27. c	137
8. b	131	28. b	138
9. a	130	29. d	133
10. d	131	30. b	138
11. c	131	31. d	138
12. a	132	32. c	139
13. c	132	33. a	139
14. d	132	34. c	140
15. a	133	35. b	141
16. b	133	36. d	141
17. c	133	37. a	141
18. d	134	38. c	141
19. c	134	39. a	142
20. a	133	40. b	142
21. b	135	41. a	144
22. c	136	42. c	150
23. d	137	43. d	149
24. d	137	44. c	134
25. b	137	45. a	136
26. a	137		

CHAPTER 8: NAIL STRUCTURE AND GROWTH

ANSWER KEY AND CORE BOOK PAGE REFERENCES

QUESTION	PAGE	QUESTION	PAGE
1. a	154	23. d	156
2. b	154	24. d	156
3. d	154	25. b	157
4. b	154	26. a	157
5. c	154	27. d	157
6. a	154	28. a	157
7. d	154	29. c	157
8. c	154	30. b	157
9. a	154	31. d	157
10. d	155	32. c	157
11. b	155	33. d	157
12. c	155	34. a	157
13. b	155	35. d	157
14. d	155	36. b	158
15. c	155	37. c	158
16. b	155	38. d	158
17. a	155	39. c	158
18. c	155	40. a	154
19. a	156	41. c	154
20. b	156	42. b	154
21. d	157	43. a	157
22. d	156	44. d	158

CHAPTER 9: NAIL DISORDERS AND DISEASES

ANSWER KEY AND CORE BOOK PAGE REFERENCES

QUESTION	PAGE	QUESTION	PAGE
1. c	162	24. b	166
2. b	162	25. b	167
3. c	162	26. d	167
4. a	163	27. c	166
5. d	165	28. a	168
6. b	165	29. c	168
7. a	163	30. b	168
8. c	163	31. a	168
9. b	163	32. c	169
10. d	163	33. b	169
11. a	163	34. d	170
12. b	163	35. a	168
13. d	163	36. b	170
14. c	163	37. a	169
15. d	164	38. c	170
16. a	164	39. b	168
17. b	164	40. d	170
18. d	164	41. c	170
19. c	164	42. a	170
20. a	164	43. b	165
21. d	165	44. d	164
22. b	165	45. c	165
23. a	166		

CHAPTER 10: THE BASICS OF CHEMISTRY

ANSWER KEY AND CORE BOOK PAGE REFERENCES

QUESTION	PAGE	QUESTION	PAGE
1. c	174	16. a	177
2. b	174	17. d	177
3. a	174	18. b	178
4. c	174	19. c	178
5. d	175	20. b	179
6. a	175	21. a	179
7. d	175	22. d	176
8. b	175	23. b	180
9. a	175	24. c	180
10. b	175	25. b	180
11. c	175	26. a	181
12. d	175	27. b	181
13. c	176	28. c	182
14. a	176	29. a	182
15. b	176	30. c	182

QUESTION	PAGE	QUESTION	PAGE
31. d	182	39. b	183
32. d	182	40. d	184
33. a	183	41. b	184
34. d	183	42. a	180
35. c	183	43. b	175
36. a	183	44. b	175
37. c	183	45. c	182
38. b	183		

CHAPTER 11: NAIL PRODUCT CHEMISTRY SIMPLIFIED

ANSWER KEY AND CORE BOOK PAGE REFERENCES

QUESTION	PAGE	QUESTION	PAGE
1. a	188	24. a	193
2. d	188	25. d	193
3. d	188	26. c	193
4. d	188	27. b	193
5. a	189	28. b	193
6. b	189	29. a	194
7. c	189	30. d	194
8. d	189	31. a	194
9. a	189	32. c	194
10. c	190	33. d	194
11. b	190	34. b	195
12. a	190	35. c	195
13. d	190	36. d	195
14. b	190	37. a	195
15. c	191	38. a	188
16. a	191	39. c	196
17. c	191	40. b	196
18. d	191	41. a	196
19. a	191	42. d	196
20. b	191	43. c	197
21. d	191	44. b	197
22. c	193	45. d	198
23. b	193		

CHAPTER 12: THE BASICS OF ELECTRICITY

ANSWER KEY AND CORE BOOK PAGE REFERENCES

QUESTION	PAGE	QUESTION	PAGE
1. c	203	7. b	203
2. d	203	8. c	203
3. a	203	9. d	203
4. b	203	10. a	203
5. b	203	11. b	204
6. d	203	12. c	204

13. d	204	30. d	207
14. b	204	31. a	207
15. a	204	32. b	207
16. d	204	33. d	207
17. c	204	34. b	208
18. a	205	35. a	207
19. b	205	36. c	208
20. b	204	37. a	208
21. d	204	38. b	208
22. b	204	39. c	209
23. c	205	40. d	209
24. a	205	41. c	204
25. b	205	42. b	203
26. c	205	43. a	204
27. d	206	44. b	204
28. d	206	45. d	209
29. c	206		

CHAPTER 13: MANICURING

ANSWER KEY AND CORE BOOK PAGE REFERENCES

QUESTION	PAGE	QUESTION	PAGE
1. c	214	23. b	226
2. b	215	24. b	228
3. d	218	25. c	230
4. b	216	26. d	230
5. c	216	27. a	231
6. b	216	28. c	225
7. b	218	29. b	231
8. d	219	30. c	231
9. c	219	31. d	232
10. b	220	32. c	233
11. a	220	33. b	234
12. c	221	34. a	236
13. b	222	35. d	236
14. a	223	36. d	236
15. c	223	37. c	237
16. d	224	38. a	244
17. b	224	39. c	239
18. a	225	40. d	248
19. d	225	41. a	242
20. a	226	42. b	252
21. c	226	43. c	254
22. a	227		

CHAPTER 14: PEDICURING

ANSWER KEY AND CORE BOOK PAGE REFERENCES

QUESTION	PAGE	QUESTION	PAGE
1. b	258	24. a	268
2. d	258	25. c	269
3. c	268	26. b	268
4. a	259	27. c	261
5. d	259	28. a	279
6. b	260	29. d	271
7. a	260	30. b	261
8. c	262	31. a	273
9. d	262	32. a	272
10. c	262	33. a	278
11. a	263	34. b	275
12. d	263	35. b	262
13. b	264	36. d	263
14. c	264	37. a	280
15. d	268	38. c	277
16. b	264	39. c	266
17. c	264	40. b	276
18. a	265	41. a	275
19. b	265	42. c	270
20. c	265	43. c	268
21. a	266	44. b	265
22. c	267	45. b	272
23. b	268		

CHAPTER 15: ELECTRIC FILING

ANSWER KEY AND CORE BOOK PAGE REFERENCES

QUESTION	PAGE	QUESTION	PAGE
1. a	285	16. a	289
2. c	285	17. c	290
3. a	285	18. d	290
4. b	285	19. a	290
5. a	286	20. a	291
6. c	286	21. a	291
7. b	286	22. b	291
8. d	286	23. a	292
9. d	286	24. b	292
10. b	287	25. c	290
11. c	288	26. d	292
12. a	287	27. a	292
13. c	288	28. b	293
14. b	289	29. d	293
15. d	289	30. c	293

Question	Page	Question	Page
31. b	289	39. b	299
32. a	289	40. d	299
33. c	297	41. c	299
34. b	297	42. c	299
35. d	298	43. b	300
36. a	294	44. b	301
37. c	298	45. a	302
38. a	298		

CHAPTER 16: NAIL TIPS AND WRAPS

ANSWER KEY AND CORE BOOK PAGE REFERENCES

QUESTION	PAGE	QUESTION	PAGE
1. b	307	24. b	311
2. a	307	25. c	311
3. c	312	26. a	316
4. a	308	27. d	319
5. c	308	28. a	314
6. b	308	29. d	315
7. d	308	30. b	312
8. c	308	31. c	313
9. a	308	32. b	313
10. d	309	33. d	317
11. b	309	34. b	317
12. b	309	35. c	317
13. b	309	36. a	317
14. d	309	37. c	318
15. a	309	38. b	310
16. c	309	39. c	319
17. d	310	40. a	322
18. b	310	41. d	309
19. d	310	42. c	309
20. a	316	43. b	316
21. b	311	44. a	308
22. a	310	45. d	311
23. d	311		

CHAPTER 17: MONOMER LIQUID AND POLYMER POWDER NAIL ENHANCEMENTS

ANSWER KEY AND CORE BOOK PAGE REFERENCES

QUESTION	PAGE	QUESTION	PAGE
1. b	327	6. d	328
2. c	328	7. a	329
3. c	328	8. b	329
4. d	329	9. c	329
5. a	328	10. a	329

11. d	329	31. c	335
12. c	330	32. a	335
13. b	330	33. d	335
14. c	330	34. b	335
15. a	330	35. d	335
16. d	330	36. a	336
17. c	330	37. b	336
18. b	331	38. c	338
19. a	331	39. b	338
20. d	331	40. c	339
21. a	342	41. a	339
22. d	332	42. b	341
23. b	332–333	43. a	342
24. a	333	44. d	343
25. d	333	45. a	345
26. a	333	46. c	346
27. c	334	47. b	343
28. d	334	48. a	349
29. a	336	49. d	349
30. c	336	50. b	351

CHAPTER 18: UV AND LED GELS

ANSWER KEY AND CORE BOOK PAGE REFERENCES

QUESTION	PAGE	QUESTION	PAGE
1. a	356	23. b	365
2. c	357	24. c	362
3. d	357	25. a	362
4. c	357	26. a	363
5. b	357	27. c	362
6. b	357	28. b	365
7. a	357	29. a	366
8. d	358	30. d	367
9. c	358	31. b	367
10. a	359	32. c	367
11. d	358	33. d	364
12. c	360	34. a	368
13. b	360	35. b	369
14. d	360	36. d	358
15. b	361	37. c	361
16. d	361	38. a	371
17. a	361	39. d	389
18. c	362	40. c	373
19. b	362	41. c	374
20. a	363	42. a	377
21. d	363	43. b	381
22. c	362	44. a	383

CHAPTER 19: THE CREATIVE TOUCH

ANSWER KEY AND CORE BOOK PAGE REFERENCES

QUESTION	PAGE	QUESTION	PAGE
1. b	388	24. a	392
2. a	389	25. b	392
3. d	389	26. d	393
4. b	390	27. c	393
5. b	390	28. b	399
6. a	390	29. a	393
7. d	390	30. d	396
8. b	390	31. d	396
9. c	390	32. c	397
10. a	390	33. d	397
11. d	390	34. a	397
12. b	390	35. d	397
13. c	390	36. b	399
14. a	391	37. c	399
15. b	391	38. b	402
16. d	391	39. a	403
17. c	390	40. a	403
18. a	392	41. d	403
19. b	391	42. c	404
20. c	392	43. b	404
21. d	392	44. a	414
22. c	392	45. c	415
23. b	392		

CHAPTER 20: SEEKING EMPLOYMENT

ANSWER KEY AND CORE BOOK PAGE REFERENCES

QUESTION	PAGE	QUESTION	PAGE
1. a	422	16. b	430
2. c	423	17. d	430
3. b	423	18. c	430
4. a	423	19. a	430
5. d	423	20. a	431
6. c	424	21. b	431
7. a	424	22. c	433
8. b	424	23. a	431
9. b	425	24. a	433
10. d	425	25. c	433
11. a	426	26. a	434
12. a	429	27. b	434
13. a	429	28. c	436
14. b	429	29. d	436
15. b	429	30. d	438

31. b	438	39. b	448
32. c	439	40. a	449
33. d	439	41. b	449
34. a	445	42. d	450
35. a	446	43. c	437
36. b	446	44. b	425
37. a	446	45. b	444
38. a	447		

CHAPTER 21: ON THE JOB

ANSWER KEY AND CORE BOOK PAGE REFERENCES

QUESTION	PAGE	QUESTION	PAGE
1. d	457	24. c	463
2. b	457	25. a	463
3. c	457	26. a	463
4. d	457	27. d	464
5. a	458	28. d	468
6. b	458	29. d	468
7. d	459	30. c	468
8. c	459	31. a	469
9. c	459	32. b	469
10. b	460	33. d	469
11. d	460	34. b	470
12. a	462	35. a	470
13. d	462	36. b	472
14. b	462	37. d	472
15. c	468	38. b	474
16. a	462	39. d	474
17. d	462	40. a	474
18. b	462	41. c	474
19. d	463	42. b	472
20. c	462	43. a	475
21. d	463	44. b	476
22. a	465	45. c	476
23. d	463		

CHAPTER 22: THE SALON BUSINESS

ANSWER KEY AND CORE BOOK PAGE REFERENCES

QUESTION	PAGE	QUESTION	PAGE
1. c	481	7. a	483
2. c	481	8. b	483
3. a	482	9. d	486
4. d	482	10. a	486
5. b	483	11. d	486
6. c	483	12. c	486

13. b	486	30. d	491
14. a	486	31. b	492
15. b	486	32. d	492
16. a	486	33. b	492
17. a	487	34. a	493
18. d	487	35. c	494
19. c	487	36. b	495
20. a	487	37. c	495
21. b	487	38. a	496
22. d	488	39. d	496
23. a	490	40. a	496
24. c	481	41. c	497
25. b	484	42. a	497
26. c	485	43. b	498
27. c	491	44. b	499
28. a	491	45. c	500
29. b	491		

Helpful Reminders for Examination Day

The following reminders have been prepared for your benefit and will assist you in passing the state board examinations.

1. *Take the time to present a professional appearance.* This includes your clothing, personal hygiene, general health, and posture.

2. *Adopt a positive mental attitude.* Doing so will help you to overcome the nervousness often associated with taking tests and exams. It might help to remember that state board exams are not given to make candidates fail, but to do justice to all candidates using measurable and objective methods of evaluation. Testing and evaluation are vital to determining a candidate's competency for the profession.

3. *Be prepared.* Create a checklist of the supplies and tools you will need for both exams. Be guided by the candidate information that usually accompanies confirmation of the test date. Make sure you bring a photo ID for identification purposes.

4. *Be punctual.* Learn in advance how to reach the test site and allow sufficient time for travel. Being on time for the exam will alleviate some stress and make it easier to maintain a positive attitude so that you can do your best.

5. *Written or computer-based tests.* Some general reminders for written or computer-based testing include the following:
   - Be ready to begin when the signal is given by the test proctor.
   - Scan the entire test before beginning to answer the questions. Then, read each test item carefully and answer the questions consecutively whenever possible.
   - Avoid spending too much time on one test item; if in doubt, continue with the test and return to the unanswered item(s) after completing the entire test.
   - If time permits, review all your answers before submitting the completed test.

6. *Practical exams.* General reminders for practical exams include:
   - Ask questions of the examiner before the signal to begin is given. Talking is prohibited during the exam.
   - Observe all cleaning and disinfecting rules during the practical exam. The use of proper infection control methods is vital to a passing score.
   - Use only clean and disinfected tools and implements.
   - Wash your hands before beginning each service.
   - Do not put implements in pockets.
   - Do not set a tool or implement down and reuse it without cleaning and disinfecting it first.